Paraplegia - New Insights

Edited by Seyed Mansoor Rayegani

Published in London, United Kingdom

Paraplegia - New Insights
http://dx.doi.org/10.5772/intechopen.102189
Edited by Seyed Mansoor Rayegani

Contributors
Nazmin Ahmed, Md. Shahidul Islam Khan, Md. Kamrul Ahsan, Mary Hannon-Fletcher, Daniel Kerr, Adrienne McCann, María José Álvarez Pérez, Saeed Oraee-Yazdani, Roozbeh Tavanaei, Seyed Mansoor Rayegani, Mohammad Hanoun, Abdelnasser Thabit, Abdullah Hanoun

First published in London, United Kingdom, 2023 by IntechOpen
IntechOpen is the global imprint of INTECHOPEN LIMITED, registered in England and Wales, registration number: 11086078, 5 Princes Gate Court, London, SW7 2QJ, United Kingdom

British Library Cataloguing-in-Publication Data
A catalogue record for this book is available from the British Library

Additional hard and PDF copies can be obtained from orders@intechopen.com

Paraplegia - New Insights
Edited by Seyed Mansoor Rayegani
p. cm.
Print ISBN 978-1-83969-779-1
Online ISBN 978-1-83969-780-7
eBook (PDF) ISBN 978-1-83969-781-4

Meet the editor

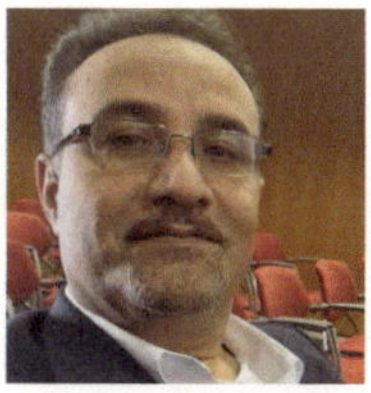

Professor S. Mansoor Rayegani heads the Physical Medicine & Rehabilitation (PM&R) Research Center at Shahid Beheshti University of Medical Sciences, Tehran, Iran, and is the Director of the Iranian PM&R board. He completed his residency training in PM&R at Shiraz University of Medical Sciences, Iran, in 1992, obtaining the top grade at the Iranian PM&R board, and became assistant professor of PM&R at Shohada Medical Center, Shahid Beheshti University of Medical Sciences in 1994. He is one of the founders of Tehran's PM&R residency training program. Professor Rayegani's interests include electrodiagnostic medicine, pain, spinal cord injury, neurorehabilitation and medical education. Supervising and coordinating electrodiagnostic medicine, neuromusculoskeletal (NMSK) pain and sono-guided injection, and neurorehabilitation clinics are among his daily professional tasks. He has supervised more than 60 postgraduate residency and fellowship theses and published about 140 indexed medical articles with 2300 citations. He is Editor in Chief of the *Journal of Physical Medicine, Rehabilitation and Electrodiagnosis (JPMRE)*, an Editorial Board member of the *Journal of the International Society of Physical and Rehabilitation Medicine (JISPRM)* and a member of the Education and Publication Committee of the ISPRM. Professor Rayegani is the current president of the Iranian PM&R Society.

Contents

Preface

Spinal cord injury with consequent catastrophic sequelae of tetraplegia and/or paraplegia is among the most debilitating medical conditions. Paraplegia is a consequence of injury to the thoracic or lumbosacral cord and/or cauda equina. The etiology of paraplegia is very important for understanding the course and prognosis of the disease and for planning treatment and rehabilitation strategies. Trauma is the most common cause of paraplegia; physical assault, car accidents, and falling are among the most frequently occurring traumatic causes. Non-traumatic causes of paraplegia are medical conditions such as multiple sclerosis, infection, nutritional deficiency, congenital processes and degenerative or inflammatory processes.

Among the concomitant and/or consequent disorders of paraplegia is pain syndrome, and for some patients, severe and intractable pain may be their main problem. Pain after paraplegia presents mainly in the lower limbs, although upper-limb pain is not uncommon in the paraplegia population. Overuse injury and repetitive traumatic injury to upper limbs during wheelchair and/or assistive device ambulation can cause upper-limb pain syndrome in paraplegia victims. In some geographic regions and countries, specific and known causes of paraplegia are present. Pott's disease is a known cause of paraplegia with a very well-documented history. Syndromes such as anterior cord syndrome, transverse myelitis and cauda equina syndrome are very common in paraplegia. Cauda equina is the involvement of multiple lumbosacral roots asymmetrically. This syndrome occurs in many circumstances such as degenerative disc disease and/or thoracolumbar acute soft disc herniation. Early detection and prompt treatment are very important in handling this potentially treatable and catastrophic condition. Like the rest of the central nervous system, the spinal cord has no post-injury regeneration capacity and tissue loss compensation. Rehabilitation medicine as a holistic approach to disability is at the heart of managing spinal cord injury and paraplegic victims.

Seyed Mansoor Rayegani, MD
Physical Medicine and Rehabilitation Research Center,
Shahid Beheshti University of Medical Sciences,
Teheran, Iran

Chapter 1

Current Etiological Profile of the Spinal Cord Injury

María José Álvarez Pérez

Abstract

The causes of spinal cord injury are multiple; classically they can be divided into two large groups: those of medical origin (tumor, infectious, vascular, by compression, sclerosis, and congenital) and those of traumatic origin (traffic accidents, accidental falls, work accidents, sports accidents (dives), attempts of autolysis, and violence). Its incidence and prevalence by sex, age, occupation, leisure activities, and geographic location are variable. The objective of this chapter is to review the different causes of spinal cord injury, especially traumatic ones, according to the different variables mentioned. The analysis of these data will allow strategies for the prevention of new injuries to be focused on the best direction.

Keywords: spinal cord injury, etiology, risk factors, SCI of medical origin, traumatic SCI

1. Introduction

Spinal cord injury (SCI) remains one of the most tragic disabilities that can happen to a person, for which there is still no regenerative or reconstructive cure. The holder of a SCI is affected with paralysis at different levels and degrees of extension, loss of sensation, and bowel, bladder, and sexual dysfunction. To this, the psychological, social, and economic consequences that this permanent physical disability involves must be added.

Spinal cord injuries are currently defined and classified according to the ASIA (American Spinal Injury Association) scale, in which a sensory and motor assessment is carried out, and a sensory, motor, and neurological level is established. This allows for homogenization of patient assessment and follow-up worldwide. It also allows to establish a prognosis, since neurological recovery is better in incomplete spinal cord injuries than in complete spinal cord injuries. Thus, different types of SCI can be distinguished according to the level, extent, and symptoms:

According to level: tetraplegia, if the paralysis affects both upper and lower limbs and paraplegia, if the paralysis only affects the lower limbs.

According to the extent: complete, when the lesion affects completely the spinal cord, and incomplete when there is a partial lesion of the spinal cord.

According to symptoms: spastic, when spasticity predominates below the level of the lesion, and flaccid, where flaccid musculature predominates below the lesion.

On the other hand, several incomplete clinical syndromes are distinguished according to their location and clinical features, such as Brown-Séquard syndrome (spinal cord hemisection), conus medullaris syndrome (sacral cord injury), and cauda equina syndrome (lumbosacral nerve root injury).

The incidence of SCI varies from country to country and among different regions. Likewise, the causes of SCI also differ from one country to another. It is therefore interesting to know these differences so that each country can work both, on treatment measures more adapted to the type of injury, above all, on prevention measures focused on working on those areas where they are most vulnerable.

1.1 Etiology of SCI

The etiology of SCI can be classically divided into two main groups: medical (or non-traumatic) and traumatic etiology.

1.2 SCI of medical origin

These represent a much lower frequency of reported cases of traumatic SCI; however, this proportion may not exactly correspond to reality due to the difficulty in recording them, which are often overlapped by the primary diseases that cause them. Thus, in Alito's study [1] with a sample of 112 patients, 76% were of non-traumatic cause, with age being significantly higher than in those of traumatic origin. With regard to age, it has been observed that in industrialized countries, the percentage of non-traumatic injuries increases together with age [2].

Something remarkable is that there is no internationally accepted term for spinal cord damage not due to trauma. Many different terms have been used in the literature to describe these conditions, including non-traumatic spinal cord injury, spinal cord damage, spinal cord dysfunction, spinal cord lesion, medical paraplegia, myelopathy, and spinal cord myelopathy [3].

The following are some of the causes of non-traumatic SCI.

1.2.1 Tumor pathology

The tumor pathology that can induce a SCI can be a primary tumor in spinal cord (ependymomas are the most common glial tumor in adults, whereas astrocytomas are the most common intramedullary tumor in children) or a metastasis. Metastatic lesions are responsible for about 85% of neoplastic spinal cord compression cases, with the other 15% due to primary neoplastic lesions of the spine [4].

Spinal cord tumors may be classified as one of two different types depending on where they occur relative to the protective membranes of the spinal cord. These are the main types of intradural tumors: intramedullary tumors (begin in the cells within the spinal cord itself, such as gliomas, astrocytomas, or ependymomas) and extramedullary tumors (grow in either the membrane surrounding the spinal cord or the nerve roots that reach out from the spinal cord, such as meningiomas, neurofibromas, schwannomas, and nerve sheath tumors). Tumors from other parts of the body can spread (metastasize) to the vertebrae, the supporting network around the spinal cord or, in rare cases, the spinal cord itself [4].

In a retrospective evaluation in a Rehabilitation Unit in the USA, between 2003 and 2014, in which they included all the patients with SCI and a diagnosis of primary or metastatic spinal cancer, most tumors were located in the thoracic region (65.4%) and were primary central nervous system in origin (21.0%), including meningioma (7.4%), schwannoma (3.7%), and ependymoma (2.5%).

The next most common origins of the spinal tumors were metastases from the lung (17.3%), prostate (9.9%), kidney (8.6%), lymphoma (7.4%), and multiple myeloma (7.4%) [5].

1.2.2 Infectious pathology

SCI of infectious origin can be caused by various etiological agents such as bacteria (tuberculosis, Mycobacterium spp), viruses (Cytomegalovirus (HCMV), Human Immunodeficiency Virus (HIV), Herpes Simplex Virus, Varicella Zoster Virus, poliovirus, HTLV-1, Zika virus), fungi (cryptococcus spp), and parasites (Toxoplasma gondii, Schistostoma mansoni).

At the National Paraplegic Hospital in Toledo (Spain), Morillo et al. [6] carried out a retrospective study of patients with SCI admitted to their center from 1997 to 2003: in the sample, infections accounted for 8% of neuropathies of medical cause, a higher figure than those reported in the classical literature. In this sample the most frequent cause of spinal cord injury was spondylodiscitis in 51% of cases followed by epidural abscesses (22.2%) and arachnoiditis (18.5%); the most frequent etiological agent was Staphilococcus Aereus in 51.9% of cases followed in frequency by Mycobacterium tuberculosis in 35.7% and brucellosis in 7.4%.

Other less frequent etiologies of SCI of infectious origin are viral infections and parasitosis, which represent 3.7% of the aforementioned sample, a figure that could increase in the coming years due to the migratory changes being experienced in Europe.

1.2.3 Rheumatological and degenerative diseases

Some rheumatological diseases such as Paget's disease, rheumatoid arthritis, osteoporosis, or the ossification of the posterior longitudinal ligament could lead to medically induced SCI.

Cervical spinal cord compression (SCC) due to degeneration of the cervical spine is a frequent finding on magnetic resonance imaging. Degenerative changes include spondylosis, degenerative disc disease, ligamental hypertrophy, and ossification of the posterior longitudinal ligament. SCC mainly occurs during later stages of life and in most cases remains asymptomatic. Nevertheless, a subset of individuals will develop symptoms, causing a condition that has recently been termed degenerative cervical myelopathy, which is the most common non-traumatic, progressive spinal cord disorder with an estimated 2% prevalence [7].

1.2.4 Inflammatory diseases

Inflammatory diseases of the nervous system, such as Multiple Sclerosis or transverse myelitis, can cause damage at different levels of the central nervous system, including the spinal cord. The exact reason for transverse myelitis is unknown, sometimes there is no known cause, and sometimes it is associated autoimmune disease. In 2021, Yu-Ting Hsiao team published a case of acute transverse myelitis after vaccination against COVID-19 with the ChAdOx1 nCOV-19 vaccine (AZD1222), which was the first case reported in Taiwan [8].

In Multiple Sclerosis, the immune system destroys the myelin that surrounds the nerves in the spinal cord and brain, and this can lead to SCI at different levels and of varying severity.

1.2.5 Neurodegenerative diseases

Degenerative diseases of the nervous system are a term used to encompass any of the diseases or disorders that are due to a loss in the function or structure of neurons of the brain or spinal cord; examples of this kind of diseases, which could cause SCI, include Lateral Amyotrophic Sclerosis (LAS), hereditary spastic paraparesis, or spinal muscular atrophy.

1.2.6 Congenital origin

There are some congenital diseases that can damage the spinal cord; some of them are cerebral palsy, diastematomelia, spinal dysraphism, Arnold-Chiari malformation, or skeletal malformations.

1.2.7 Iatrogenesis

Iatrogenesis is unintended and unwanted damage to health caused as an unavoidable side effect of an active medical act, whether diagnostic or therapeutic. SCI secondary to iatrogenesis is common, and it is expected to grow, due to the increasing life expectancy of the population, which leads to an increase in the number of elderly patients with vascular risk factors undergoing invasive interventions. It is important to take into account whether the patient with SCI has required surgery to improve their prognosis or if, on the contrary, the SCI has been produced as a consequence of a surgical act.

In the study carried out by Montalva Iborra [9], the 18.18% of a sample of 265 patients with acute SCI were caused by iatrogenesis; the most frequent level of injury was the thoracic level (48%), and the main etiology was surgery for degenerative spine disease, where patients under the age of 30 were treated with intrathecal chemotherapy. The SCI rising during anesthetic practice is a rare event, which could be produced by direct (e.g., spinal nerve root damage due to incorrect pedicle screw placement) or indirect (e.g., cord ischemia following aortic surgery) factors [10].

1.2.8 Other causes of non-traumatic SCI

Other non-traumatic causes of SCI are *vascular causes* (spinal cord infarction), *post-injury sequelae*, such as Syrigomyelia, *toxic causes*, as radiation or chemotherapy, and *genetical and metabolic disorders,* such as vitamin B12 deficiency or abetalipoproteinemia.

The medical causes of SCI are included in **Table 1** [11].

1.3 Traumatic SCI

Traumatic cause is the most epidemiologically significant etiology, with a frequency ranging from 66 to 87% of all reported cases of SCI, according to ASPAYM (**Table 2**) [11].

It should be noted that the etiology of the injury is usually associated with the level, so that the majority of sports injuries, falls, and approximately 50% of traffic accidents correspond to the cervical level [12].

Tumor pathology	Primary tumor or metastases (intra and extramedullary).
Infectious pathology	Bacterial cause: Pott's disease (tuberculosis), mycobacterium spp. Myelitis of viral etiology: Cytomegalovirus (HCMV), Human Immunodeficiency Virus (HIV), herpes simplex virus, varicella zoster virus, poliovirus, HTLV-1. Mycosis: cryptococcus spp. Parasite: toxoplasma gondii, Schistostoma mansoni.
Rheumatological and degenerative diseases	Spondylosis, stenosis, disc pathology, Paget's disease, rheumatoid arthritis, osteoporosis, ossification of the posterior longitudinal ligament.
Inflammatory diseases	Multiple Sclerosis, transverse mielitis.
Neurodegenerative disorders	Lateral Amiotrophic Sclerosis; Hereditary spastic paraparesis; Spinal muscular atrophy.
Congenital origin	Cerebral palsy, diastematomelia,...
Vascular	Spinal cord infarct
Iatrogenesis	Spinal taps, epidural catheter placement, aortic repair...
Post-injury sequelae	Syringomyelia
Toxic causes	Radiation, chemotherapy.
Genetical and metabolical disorders	Vitamin B12 deficiency, abetalipoproteinemia.

Table 1.
Medical causes of SCI.

Traffic accidents	Car accidents, motorcycle accidents, collision/knocking down.
Casual falls	From great height, from own height.
Accidents at work	Accidents with heavy machinery, falls...
Sports accidents /Recreative activities	Diving. Skiing. Horse riding. Contact sports (rugby, American football). Extreme sports (skydiving, paragliding).
Attempted self-injury	Suicide attempted
Others	Violence (firearms injuries, stab wounds, direct traumas). Electrical injuries.

Table 2.
Traumatic causes of SCI.

On the other hand, there are factors that increase the risk of SCI related to living conditions [12]; thus, the type of work activity, its category and the sector where it is carried out have a great influence on the incidence of SCI. Some jobs carry a higher risk of traumatic SCI. This is to some extend related to socioeducational variables, as some of the jobs with the highest risk of injury are often those with the lowest educational requirements. In relation to the socioeconomic situation of the place where the person lives as well as their particular conditions, the type of transport they use, the sport activities they do, and the climate of violence they may be exposed will differ.

Socioeconomic and occupational variables imply the emergence of a new profile of SCI worldwide, which takes into account the different development of each country as well as population movements, which deserve a detailed analysis.

2. Materials and methods

2.1 Design

This is a literature review in which a search for publications on etiology of traumatic and non-traumatic SCI worldwide has been carried out.

2.2 Selection criteria

Inclusion criteria: those dealing with the etiology of SCI publications within the last 30 years (due to the scarcity of publications in some geographic areas of the world) and those in English or Spanish.

Exclusion criteria: excluded epidemiological studies that did not provide a comprehensive analysis of the etiology of traumatic or non-traumatic SCI, studies without full text available and those found in other languages.

2.3 Search strategy

A bibliographic search was carried out from January 1989 to August 2022 in the following database: PubMed and Cochrane. The following keywords were used: spinal cord injury, traumatic, non-traumatic, etiology, epidemiology. A combination of these terms was used thanks to the Boolean operator "and" and "or."

3. Results and discussion

A total of 58 documents were reviewed, of which 50 were scientific articles according to the inclusion and exclusion criteria mentioned in the previous section. In addition, a doctoral thesis, a paper of a conference, a reference of three books, two web pages, and an informative guide were included, all of which were referenced in one of the articles reviewed.

The results found are collected discussed below, separated by non-traumatic and traumatic etiology as well as by geographical area.

3.1 Non-traumatic SCI

3.1.1 Results

The etiology of non-traumatic SCI was reviewed worldwide by New PW[13], which included the abstracts of 377 publications and 45 reports from 24 countries in 12 of the 21 WHO global regions. The results were the following:

3.1.1.1 Asia

Pacific Asia presented a high rate of degenerative deformity of the spine (59%) and tumors (19%). South Asia (India) showed a high rate of tuberculosis (38–25%), followed by tumors.

3.1.1.2 Australia

Tumors, degenerative and vascular conditions were the main causes of non-traumatic SCI.

3.1.1.3 Europe

Western Europe presented high rates of tumors and degenerative conditions (25% and 32% medians, respectively), quite likely influenced by the age profile of the western European population. Spina bifida was reported as a cause of non-traumatic SCI in Spain, Italy (both 5%), and Denmark (2%). Myelitis was lower in Israel (7%) and higher in Denmark (14%) and Italy (23%).

3.1.1.4 Africa

In north Africa/middle east, spinal tumors and degenerative causes of non-traumatic SCI were the most commonly diagnosed conditions. Tumors and degenerative conditions were slightly higher in Ankara (29% for both causes) than in Istanbul (22% and 25%, respectively). Inflammatory conditions were common in Ankara (23%) and in Istanbul (20%). Six percentage of non-traumatic SCI cases reported in Istanbul were spina bifida.

In east sub-Saharan Africa, tuberculosis was a major cause: this etiology was highest in Kenya and Malawi (33% in both countries) and lower in Ethiopia (20 and 27%). HIV-related non-traumatic SCI was common in Ethiopia (17%) and was not reported in Kenya or Malawi. Tumor-related non-traumatic SCI cases were highest in Kenya (33%), Malawi (25%), and Ethiopia (22%). Myelitis was low in Ethiopia (4%) and Malawi (7%).

In southern sub-Saharan Africa, tumors and tuberculosis-related non-traumatic SCI cases were high (28% and 27%, respectively). Transverse myelopathy accounted for 11% of the non-traumatic SCI cases.

In west sub-Saharan Africa, tuberculosis was relatively common in both Ghana and Nigeria (30% and 25%, respectively), and the proportion of neoplastic SCI and myelitis was similar in both countries (about 15% and 12%, respectively).

3.1.1.5 America

According to literature, in North America, spinal stenosis and tumors were common (54% and 26%, respectively) and myelitis was low (5%).

3.1.1.6 Oceania

In Oceania, the most frequent cause of non-traumatic SCI was infection (32%), and tumors only represented 9%.

An overview of the etiology of non-traumatic SCI can be seen in **Figure 1**, extracted from New PW [13].

3.1.2 Discussion

There tended to be more reports of better quality from high-income countries compared with medium- and low-income countries [13]. Developed countries tended

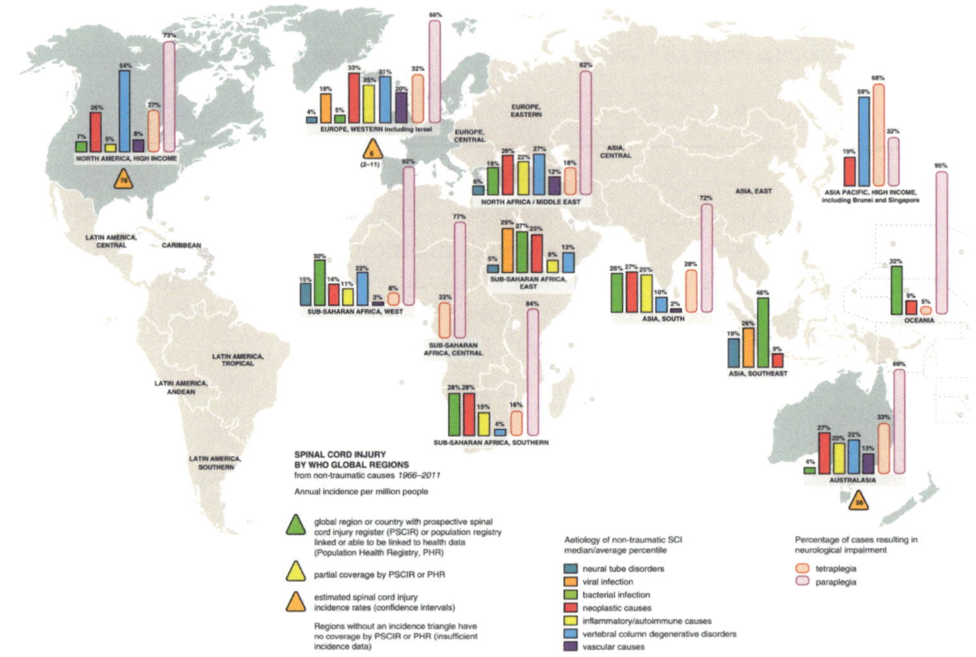

Figure 1.
Global maps of NTSCI epidemiological outcomes (1959–2011) by WHO global regions [13].

to have a higher proportion of cases with degenerative conditions and tumors causing SCI [11]. Developing countries, in comparison, tended to have a higher proportion of infections, particularly tuberculosis and HIV, although it was interesting that a number also reported tumors as a major cause [13].

3.2 Traumatic SCI

3.2.1 Results

The different *causes of traumatic SCI* vary greatly in incidence and prevalence from country to country and are discussed in detail below according to the various published studies.

In *developing countries*, motor vehicle collisions were the cause of traumatic SCI in 41% of cases, followed by falls in 34.8%, although there are differences between countries that will be discussed below, according Rahimi-Movaghar's review (**Table 3**) [14].

In countries such as Bangladesh, where urbanization and motorization are less developed, falls remain the leading cause (63%), related to fruit picking and loading as part of agricultural practice, rather than osteoporosis as in developed countries. This is also the case in Pakistan (82% due to falls from trees or roofs) and Nepal (61%) [15]; in both countries road traffic accidents account for around 7% of traumatic SCI [16–18].

However, in Vietnam and Thailand, transport accidents are the leading cause (47%), most of them involving motorbikes, as they are the main means of transport [15]. In 31 of the studies analyzed by Rahimi-Movaghar [14], road traffic crashes were

Country	First author	Motor vehicle	Fall	Gunshot wound	Violence	Sport
Bangladesh	Hoque et al., 1999	18	63			
Brazil	Brito et al., 2011 Barros Filho et al., 1990	41.4 26.9	42.6 22.4		36,.7	7.9
China	Ning et al., 2011	34.1	56.9		1.4	0.2
India	Manjeet et al., 2009	30.3	50		2.7	0.7
Russia	Kondakov et al., 2002	16	34			2
Sudáfrica	Velmahos et al., 1995 Hart y Williams, 1994	30 28	3	61 62		
Irán	Rahimi-Movaghar et al., 2009	64	12			
Nigeria	Obalum et al., 2009	77.4	9.4	7.3	2.1	1.7

Table 3.
Etiology of traumatic SCI in developing countries (table extracted from Rahimi-Movaghar et al., 2013) [14].

more frequent, and in one, both causes had similar percentages. Thus, in two studies from Nigeria and one from Saudi Arabia, motor vehicle collision accounted for more than 80% of cases [14].

In two studies from South Africa, with more than 50% of the cases, and in one from Brazil, violence was the first cause. In South Africa, the etiology has shifted from stab wound (38% in 1998 to 17.5% in 1992) to firearm (28.5% in 1988 to 47% in 1992) as the most frequent cause, with only 3% fall injuries [19].

In the Nigerian city of Plateau, in contrast, tunnel collapse in illegal mines was the most prevalence cause [14]. However, in a hospital in Enugu, Nigeria, the most cause of traumatic SCI in their sample was car accident (55.3%), with a decrease in injuries caused by falling from a palm tree from 40.2% of SCI in 1988 to 3.5% [20].

In Rahimi's systematic review [14], an annual increase of 0.9% in the relative frequency of traumatic SCI-related falls was detected during the study period between 1975 and 2009. Male gender, age, or type of complete or incomplete injury and neurological damage (tetraplegia or paraplegia) showed no association with mechanism of injury in these countries [14]. Etiologies were also studied by groups or seasons; in India, an increase in injuries was detected during the summer period, related to an increase in population movements during this period, with injuries being more frequent in natives than in visitors to the country, and Nigeria recorded the highest peaks of SCI during the celebration of the most important festivals [20].

Other articles published between 2011 and 2013 that were not included in the Rahimi-Movaghar systematic review are listed below. In the Emergency Unit of

Haydarpasa Hospital in Ankara, falls from height (50.6%) represent the first cause of traumatic SCI, associated with lumbar injuries, followed by falls from small heights (20.8%), more related to thoracic injuries [21]. On the other hand, a clear relationship was observed between traffic accidents and cervical (p = 0.00001) and lumbar injuries (p = 0.004) and sports accidents and cervical injuries (p = 0.014). The season with the highest number of injuries was summer [21].

In Anhui province in China [22], the leading cause in the sample of 761 traumatic SCI patients analyzed was fall from height (52.6%) in both men and women, followed by road traffic accidents (21.2%), something also observed in Tianjin [23], where a review of cervical SCI was conducted, with 49.7% of injuries caused by falls (an increase in incidence in low falls and a decrease in high falls with age), and 36.4% by traffic, while in Mainland [24], in the same country, in a review of 82.720 patients, the majority of traumatic SCI was caused by motor vehicle accidents (33.61%), closely followed by falls from height (31.25%) and trivial falls (23.23%). A subsequent study in Guangdong province (China) has shown an increase in the number of people suffering from SCI and a rising trend; the leading causes were falls and motor vehicles collisions. The low-falls (height < 1 m) group has expanded over this period, related to population aging [25].

In contrast, in Malaysia, in the review conducted at Kuala Lumpur Hospital between 2006 and 2009, 66% of traumatic SCI cases were caused by motor vehicle accidents and 28% by falls [26].

In Jordan, the leading cause is four-wheeled vehicle accidents, related to high speed and lack of seat belts, but not alcohol, given the high percentage of Muslims; in this country, accidental gunshots account for 26% [15].

In Turkey, road traffic accidents account for almost half of the cases (49%), followed by falls (37%) from trees and roof (more in the summer months, when people sleep on roofs), mainly among children and elderly people [15].

In Central and South America, information is only available from Brazil: road accidents account for 35% of traumatic SCI, more frequent in cars than on motorbikes; those related to violence, specifically gunshot wounds, account for 30% of cases [15]. However, in the study conducted at the UFMA University Hospital in the state of Maranhao in Brazil, between January 2008 and June 2009, falls accounted for 42.6%, traffic 41.4%, gunshot wounds 12.6%, and dives 3.4% [27].

In *developed countries*, road traffic accidents continue to be the most frequent cause of traumatic SCI, although their proportion, especially in young men, has decreased in recent years with respect to falls, especially in older people, and even non-traumatic SCI. The results are broken down by continent.

3.2.1.1 Asia

The review carried out at the Yunsel University College of Medicine Hospital in Seoul between 2004 and 2008 places car accidents as the leading cause of traumatic SCI, with a statistically significant increase in injuries caused by falls, and a decrease in those caused by firearm or penetrating wounds. Likewise, there is a decrease in traumatic SCI with an increase in non-traumatic SCI (traumatic causes represented between 1987 and 1996 91.2% and between 2004 and 2008 76.5% [28]).

In Japan, falls account for 42% of cases, which is probably related to an aging population [29, 30].

3.2.1.2 North America

In the 2005–2011 review of SCI of any etiology collected in NSCID and NSSCID, two SCI databases in the USA, the most frequent causes of SCI were car accidents (31.5%) and falls (25.3%), followed by firearms injuries (10.4%), motorbike accidents (6.8%), diving accidents (4.7%), and those due to medical or surgical complications (4.3%) [31]. Road traffic accidents remain the leading cause of SCI in the USA, although the percentage of injuries caused by falls increased from 17% in the 1970s to 28% in 2005–2011 [32]. There has been a little change in SCI caused by motor vehicle accidents: in the 1970s, the motor vehicle etiology accounted for 47.6% and in 2000 48.3% [33]. In a review conducted at a major trauma center in California between 1996 and 2008, 32.6% of traumatic SCI cases were caused by motor vehicle accidents; although traffic accidents were also the leading cause in this study, a decrease was noted, which was related to improved vehicle safety and traffic regulations [34].

In the United States, SCI caused by violence increase by 29% between 1973 and 1999, with a significant decrease (14%) after 2000, values that are well above those reported in Western Europe and Australia, being a frequent etiology in urban settings in developed countries [30]. DeVivo [33, 35], analyzing NSCISC data, notes that acts of violence, specified as firearm injuries, constitute the third leading cause of SCI globally, at 17%.

Sport or recreationally motivated SCI is on the other hand decreasing (from 14% in 1970s to 8% between 2005 and 2011 [31] and from 14.2% in 1970s to 10% in 2000 [33]. Injury prevention initiatives have reduced cases of SCI, such as diving, American football, or trampoline jumping; however, they are increasing in relation to winter sports [33]. In the USA, diving ranks fourth in frequency with 7.3%, behind violent acts [34]. These percentages are very variable when comparing different countries [22, 36–38]: Russia with 23%, Poland with 19.8%, Australia 10.4%, Brazil with 9.3%, or the state of Florida in the USA with 8.5%.

In Canada [39], very similar percentages were found for motor vehicle collision (35%) and falls (31%), the latter being the leading cause in people over 60 (57%) and even more so in those over 80 (89%), which is consistent with other publications where falls are the leading cause of traumatic SCI in women over 60 and men over 70 [40].

3.2.1.3 Europe

Data on traumatic SCI in Europe also varies from one country to another.

In Estonia, according to Saber's study [41], 41% of traumatic SCI cases were caused by falls, which were the most frequently recorded etiology in the over 30 age group (thus, above the age of 60, accounting for 72.4% of traumatic SCI) and only 29% were caused by road traffic accidents, which proved to be the most frequent cause below the age of 30. Alcohol consumption preceded such injuries in 43.2% of cases.

In a study conducted in Oslo [42], in which only traumatic cervical fractures were studied, 60% of them were caused by falls, more associated with older people, 21% were caused by car accidents, 8% were associated with cycling, and 4% with diving, the latter being more frequent in younger people.

In Iceland, the most frequent cause of SCI is traffic accident: Knutsdottir et al. [43] reported 42.5% of traumatic SCI caused by road traffic accidents, most of which were associated with non-use of seat belts; the second cause was falls with 30.9% with an increase in falls from height in the elderly group, associated with cervical injuries and incompleteness. Sports accounted for 18.8%, related to horse riding and winter sports, especially in the female group [42].

In Poland [44] and Romania [45], road traffic accidents are the first cause, as in the rest of Western European countries.

Bicycle accidents are highly representative in the Netherlands, Greece, Denmark, and Ireland [15]; motorbike accidents are more frequent in Greece and Italy compared with other European countries.

Given that Europe has a high proportion of people over 60 years of age, falls account for 32% of traumatic SCI in Western Europe.

SCI related to self-harm attempts varies from 1 to 26% with an average of 8%: thus, Scandinavian countries have a high suicide rate, where only intentional precipitation accounts for 8% of all cases of traumatic SCI [36]. Greenland (Denmark) has the highest rate of all: 15% of traumatic SCI cases are caused by accidental shooting, according to Pedersen et al. [46]; on the other hand, transport accidents, especially motorbike accidents, account for 4%, the lowest figure of all articles reviewed, as do skiing accidents (4%); 50% of all SCI occur under the influence of alcohol [46].

Riding-related SCI cases are highest in Ireland, Switzerland, and Iceland [15].

In Spain, between 2000 and 2008 (Working Group of the Spanish Society of Epidemiology, 2011), 50% of cases were caused by a traffic accident, 20–30% by a casual fall, 8% by an accident at work, 4–11% by sport or leisure activity, and 1% by violence. Traffic accidents are therefore the leading cause of traumatic SCI in this country, and of these, those produced in four-wheeled vehicles are the most common. Mazaira's team [47] related it to 52.4% of the total traumatic etiology and García Reneses [48, 49] to 45%. According to the latter author, 84% occur in four-wheeled vehicles, 9.6% in two-wheeled vehicles, and 6.4% in pedestrians. In those produced in four-wheeled vehicles, 58.2% affected drivers and 41.8% affected passengers, although it was not differentiated whether the passengers occupied the front or rear passenger seat. There was a significant increase in the incidence of traumatic SCI with road traffic accident etiology and a predominance of males, with a Male/Female ratio greater than 4 [47]. During the last decades, safety measures have been implemented, many of them aimed at increasing the severity of traffic laws. The second most frequent cause was falls from height, casual falls, and falls at work. In the study carried out in eight Spanish autonomous communities [47], casual falls accounted for 22.8%, more related to advanced age, and work-related falls accounted for 13.6%; these data coincide with those found in the Canary Islands [50], where the occupational accident was also assessed in isolation and related to the etiology. In Aragon [51], falls account 24.6% of traumatic SCI, a figure that is increasing while traffic accidents causing this type of injury are decreasing, with the highest number of cases found in the second decade of life in women, and fifth and eighth in both sexes. In terms of sporting etiology, most of them occur in people under 30 years of age. In Van den Berg's study [52], it accounted for 1.9% behind violent causes, while Mazaira and his team [47] put it at third place with 5.3%, with diving being the main etiology in all the studies reviewed, a figure that coincides with those provided for the Canary Islands (10.4% of all traumatic etiologies are due to diving) [50]. The study by Alén Garabato [53] examines diving as a significant etiology in this country between 1974 and 1995; it is the fifth cause of SCI, with 3.4% of all injuries. Of all those affected, 87.7% were under 30 years of age, with a distribution of 76.5% on beaches, 21.5% in swimming pools, and 2% in lakes. Cervical injuries accounted for 98% of the injuries, with summer being the season with the highest incidence. Data on SCI secondary to violence are scare with ranging from 0.95% [39], 1.3% [47], 1.8% [50] to 3.9% [53].

All these results are below those found in other studies in developed countries, such as the United States. The data found for international falls from height, or precipitation, are variable: in the Canary Islands, it is 2.8% [51]; in the ASPAYM's study, it is 2.5% [13]; and in the Mazaira study [47], it is 2.3%, all of them below 8% of the Nordic countries, which have the highest figures in Europa.

3.2.1.4 Oceania

In Australia [54] and New Zealand [55], the leading cause of traumatic SCI is road traffic accidents due to motor vehicles; SCI of sporting etiology is approximately 3% more frequent in New Zealand, with rugby accounting for 8% of all those in this category. In both, falls account for a quarter and a third of all traumatic SCI, respectively.

In the Fiji Islands, falls account for 39% followed by sports (28%); road accidents account for no more than 25% [56].

3.2.2 Discussion

The most common etiologies in developing countries are road traffic accidents and falls from height. Both of them are increasing due to urbanization and increased use of motor vehicles; the WHO foresees a further growth in traumatic SCI due to road traffic accidents if preventive measures are not put in place. In contrast, in developed countries, although road traffic accidents continue to be the most frequent cause of traumatic SCI, this proportion is decreasing due to an increase in falls, especially in older people, as well as an increase in non-traumatic etiology.

Figure 2 provides an overview of the etiology of both traumatic and non-traumatic SCI worldwide from the Lancet 2019 [57].

3.3 Analysis of the etiology in terms of age

The etiology profile was analyzed *by age group* by Price [58]: motor vehicle collision is the leading cause in the USA up to the age of 45 years, and above this, falls (75% of the cases recorded in people aged 76 years and over, are caused by falls). Between the ages of 16 and 30, firearm injury ranks second (19%) and third between the ages of 10 and 15 (8.1%), with this etiology declining as the age of the persons affected increases. Motorbike accidents represent the third most frequent cause between 31 and 45 years (10.9%) and 46–60 years (7.1%). Medical-surgical complications are the second most frequent cause under the age of 16 (12.8%) and the third most frequent cause over the age of 60 (10.9%).

If one looks only at what happens in childhood [3], non-traumatic SCI was mostly due to tumors (30–63%) and inflammatory/autoimmune causes (28–35%), and traumatic SCI was mostly caused by land transport (46–74%), falls (12–35%), and sport or recreation (10–25%) .

3.4 Analysis of the etiology in terms of sex

Analyzing the etiology *according to sex*, the two main causes of SCI, car accidents and falls, accounted for 53.5% of the total among males and 68.6% among females, while firearm injuries (11.7% in males and 5.8% in females), motorbike accidents (8% in males and 2.4% in females), or dives (5.3% in males and 2.4% in females) were more numerous among males. In contrast, medical-surgical complications

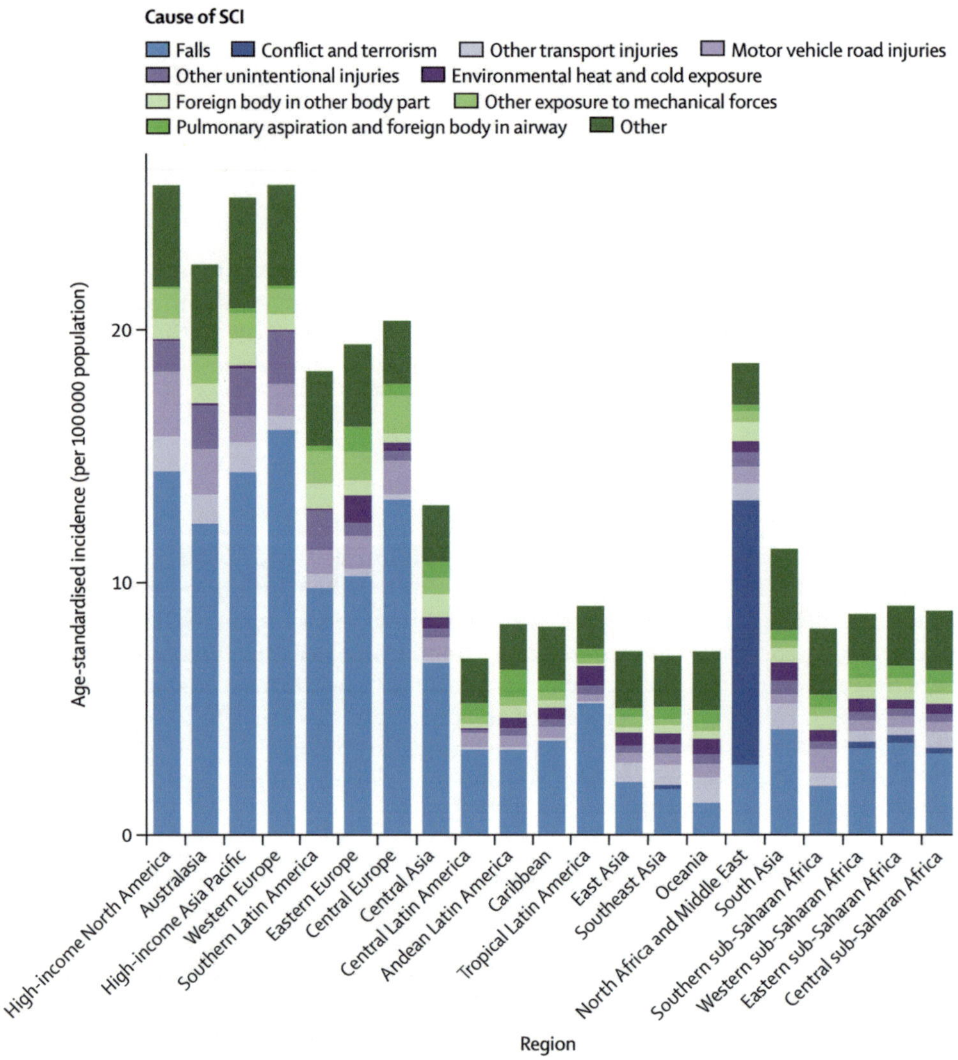

Figure 2.
An overview of the etiology of SCI [57].

represent the third cause of SCI in women (7.6%) and the sixth among men (3.3%), according to Price [58].

3.5 Analysis of the etiology in terms of ethnicity

Price et al. pointed out that the largest differences in the etiological profile were found in the *ethnicity*: firearm injuries caused 33% of SCI in blacks, 14.6% in Hispanics, 9.5% in other races, and only 3% in whites [58].

3.6 Analysis of the etiology in terms of temporality

There are notable differences between the days of the week and the season in which most traumatic and non-traumatic SCIs occur. On the one hand, most traumatic SCI takes place on weekends: Price et al. [58] found that most SCI occurred on Saturday (18.9%) and Sunday (17.3%), which is explained by the higher number of motorbike accidents and dives during the *weekend*; in contrast, medical-surgical complications are more frequent on Monday or Tuesday (19.8% and 21% respectively).

On the other hand, the month with the highest number of SCI was July (10.9%), compared with February (6.3%), which was the lowest, which is also related to the increased use of water sports and motorbikes in the warmer months [58].

3.7 Relationship between etiology and type of SCI

The level and complexity (complete and incomplete) of the injury were associated with the etiology: firearms injuries and medical-surgical complications result in paraplegia, especially at the D7-S3 level [58]. In contrast, falls generally result in tetraplegia [57]. A large number of falls and medical-surgical complications result in incomplete injuries, while firearm and motorbike injuries result in complete injuries [58].

4. Conclusions

A more comprehensive understanding of the epidemiology of SCI is required to better plan health services that can meet the future demand for prevention and rehabilitation of people with spinal cord damage from any cause.

4.1 Limitations

A limitation of this review is that there is a scarcity of quality research in the field of SCI epidemiology; most studies are single-center, with the potential for selection bias to influence the results. Furthermore, there was no internationally accepted classification of non-traumatic SCI available at the time that the studies included in this review were carried out. This limited the ability to report and compare the etiology across many countries and regions.

Author details

María José Álvarez Pérez
Independent Researcher, Madrid, Spain

*Address all correspondence to: draalvarezrehabilitacion@gmail.com

References

[1] Alito B, Filardi V, Famà F, Bruschetta D, Ruggeri C, Basile G, et al. Traumatic and non-traumatic spinal cord injury: Demographic characteristics, neurological and functional outcomes. A 7-year single centre experience. Journal of Orthopaedics. 2021;**28**:62-66

[2] Rupp R. Spinal Cord lesions. Handbook of Clinical Neurology. 2020;**168**:51-65

[3] New PW, PW. A narrative Review of Pediatric Nontraumatic Spinal Cord Dysfunction. Topics in Spinal Cord Injury Rehabilitation. 2019;**25**(2): 112-120. Spring

[4] Mayo Clinic [Internet]. Spinal Cord Tumor. Mayo Clinic Org. [date of consultation 8.23.2022]. Avalaible at: https://www.mayoclinic.org/diseases-conditions/spinal-cord-tumor/symptoms-causes/syc-20350103

[5] Ge L, Karan A, Ikpeze T, Baldwin A, Nickels JL, Mesfin A. Traumatic and Nontraumatic Spinal Cord Injuries. World Neurosurgery. 2018;**111**:142-148

[6] Morillo-LecoG,Alcaraz-RousseletMA, Díaz-Borrego P, Sáenz-Ramírez L, ArtimeC,Labarta-BertolC.Características clínicas de la lesión medular de causa infecciosa. Revista de Neurologia. 2005;**41**(4):205-208

[7] Smith SS, Stewart ME, Davies BM, Kotter MRN. The Prevalence of of Asymptomatic and Symptomatic Spinal Cord Compression on Magnetic Resonance Imaging: A Systematic Review and Meta-analysis. Global Spine Journal. 2021;**11**(4):597-607

[8] Hsiao Y-T, Tsai M-J, Chen Y-H, Hsu C-F. Acute transverse myelitis after COVID-19 Vaccination. Medicina (Kaunas, Lithuania). 2021;**57**(10):1010

[9] Montalva-Iborra A, Alcanyis-Alberola M, Grao-Castellote C, Torralba-Collados F, Giner-Pascual M. Risk factors in iatrogenic spinal cord injury; some of them are directly related with the technic. Spinal Cord. 2017;**55**(9):818-822

[10] Hewson DW, Bedforth NM, Hardman JG. Spinal cord injury airsing in anaesthesia practice. Anaesthesia. 2018;**73**(Suppl. 1):43-50

[11] Strassburguer Lona K, Hernández Porras Y, Barquín SE. Guía para el manejo integral del paciente con lesión medular crónica. Madrid: ASPAYM Madrid; 2013

[12] ASPAYM. Análisis sobre la Lesión Medular en España. Informe de Resultados [Internet]. Toledo: Federación Nacional ASPAYM; 2009 [date of consultation 8.23.2022]. Avalaible at: www.aspaym.org

[13] New PW, Cripps RA, Bone LB. Global maps of non-traumatic spinal cord injury epidemiology: towards a living data repository. Spinal Cord. 2014;**52**(2):97-109

[14] Rahimi-Movaghar V, Sayyah MK, Akbari H, Khorramirouz R, Rasouli MR, Moradi-Lakeh M, et al. Epidemiology of traumatic spinal cord injury in developing countries: a systematic review. Neuroepidemiology. 2013;**41**:65-85

[15] Cripps RA, Lee BB, Wing P, Weerts E, Mackay J, Brown D. A global map of traumatic spinal cord injury epidemiology: towards a living data

repository forinjury prevention. Spinal Cord. 2011;**49**:493-501

[16] Raja IA, Vohra AH, Ahmed M. Neurotrauma in Pakistan. World Journal of Surgery. 2001;**25**:1230-1237

[17] Lakhey S, Jha N, Shrestha BP, Niraula S. A etioepidemiological profile of spinal cord injury patients in Eastern Nepal. Tropical Doctor. 2005;**35**:231-233

[18] Hagen EM, Rekand T, Gilhus NE, Gronning M. Traumatic spinal cord injuries: incidence, mechanisms and course. Tidsskrift for den Norske Lægeforening. 2012;**132**:831-837

[19] Hart C, Williams E. Epidemiology of spinal cord injuries: a reflection of changes in South African society. Paraplegia. 1994;**32**:709-714

[20] Nwankwo OE, Uche EO. Epidemiological and treatment profiles of spinal cord injury insoutheast Nigeria. Spinal Cord. 2013;**51**(6):448-452

[21] Erdogan MÖ, Anlas Demir S, Kosargelir M, Colak S, Öztürk E. Local differences in the epidemiology of traumatic spinal injuries. Ulusal Trauma ve Acil Cerrahi Dergisi. 2013;**19**:49-52

[22] Wang HF, Yin ZS, Chen Y, Duan ZH, Hou S, He J. Epidemiological features of traumatic spinal cord injury in Anhui Provence, China. Spinal Cord. 2013;**51**:20

[23] Wu Q, Li Y, Ning G-Z, Feng S-Q, Chu T-C, Li Y, et al. Epidemiology of traumatic cervical spinal cord injuryin Tianjin, China. Spinal Cord. 2012;**50**:740-744

[24] Liu P, Yao Y, Liu MY, Fan WL, Chao R, Wang ZG, et al. Spinal trauma in Mainland China from 2001 to 2007: an epidemiological study based on a nationwide database. Spine (Phila PAa 1976). 2012;**37**:1310-1315

[25] Chen J, Chen Z, Zhang H, Song D, Wang C, Xuan T. Epidemiological features of traumatic spinal cord injury in Guangdong Province, China. Journal of Spinal Cord Medicine. 2021;**44**(2):276-281

[26] Ibrahim A, Lee KY, Kanoo LL, Tan CH, Hamid MA, Hamedon NM, et al. Epidemiology of Spinal Cord Injury in Hospital Kuala Lumpur. Spine (Phila Pa 1976). 2013;**38**(5):419-424

[27] Brito LM, Chein MB, Marinho SC, Duarte TB. Epidemiological evaluation of victims of spinal cord injury. Revista do Colégio Brasileiro de Cirurgiões. 2011;**38**:304-309

[28] Cheol Shin JC, Klim DH, Yu SJ, Yang HE, Yoon SY. Epidemiologic change of patients with spinal cord injury. Annals of Rehabilitation Medicine. 2013;**37**:50-56

[29] Ide M, Ogata H, Tokuhiro A, Takechi H. Spinal cord injuries in Okayama Prefecture: an epidemiological study 88-89. Journal of UOEH. 1993;**15**(3):209-215

[30] Shingu H, Ohama M, Ikata T, Katoh S, Akatsu T. A nationwide epidemiological survey of spinal cord injuries in Japan from January 1990 to December 1992. Paraplegia. 1995;**33**:183-188

[31] Chen Y, Tang Y, Vogel LC, MJ DV. Causes of Spinal Cord Injury. Topics in Spinal Cord Injury Rehabilitation. 2013;**19**:1-8

[32] DeVivo MJ. Epidemiology of traumatic spinal cord injury: trends and future implications. Spinal Cord. 2012;**50**:365-372

[33] DeVivo MJ. Epidemiology of spinal cord injury. En: Lin VW, ed. Spinal Cord Medicine. Second Edition. New York: Demos Medical Publishing; 2010.pp. 78-84

[34] Oliver M, Inaba K, Tang A, Branco BC, Barmparas G, Schnüriger B, et al. The changing epidemiology of spinal trauma: a 13 year review from a Level I trauma centre. Injury. 2012;**43**:1296-1300

[35] DeVivo MJ. Epidemiology of traumatic spinal cord injury. En: Kishblum S, Capagnolo DI, DeLisa JA, editors. Spinal cord Medicines. Philadelphia: Lippincott Williams and Wikins; 2002. pp. 69-81

[36] Biering-Sorensen F, Pedersen V, Clausen S. Epidemiology of spinal cord lesions in Denmark. Paraplegia. 1990;**28**:105-118

[37] Al N, Go BK, Karunas RB. Recent demographic and injury trends in people served by the model spinal cord injury caresystems. Archives of Physical Medicine and Rehabilitation. 1999;**80**:1372-1382

[38] Pleguezuelos E, Pineda S, Ramirez L, Castelló T, García L. Lesión medular por arma de fuego. Las Palmas de Gran Canaria, España: XX Congreso Nacional de la Sociedad Española de Paraplejia(Ed); 2003

[39] Pickett GE, Campos-Benitez M, Keller JL, Duggal N. Epidemiology of traumatic spinal cord injury in Canada. Spine (Phila Pa 1976). 2006;**31**:799-805

[40] Dryden DM, Saunders LD, Rowe BH, May LA, Yiannakoulias N, Svenson LW, et al. The epidemiology of traumatic spinal cord injury in Alberta, Canada. The Canadian Journal of Neurological Sciences. 2003;**30**:113-121

[41] Sabre L, Pedai G, Rekand T, Asser T, Linnamägi U, KÖrv J. High incidence of traumatic spinal cord injury in Estonia. Spinal Cord. 2012;**50**:755-759

[42] FredØ HL, Rizvi SA, Lied B, RØnning P, Helseth E. The epidemiology of traumatic cervical spine fractures: a prospective population study from Norway. Scandinavian Journal of Trauma, Resuscitation and Emergency Medicine. 2012;**20**:85

[43] Knutsdottir S. Spinal cord injuries in Iceland 1973-1989.A follow up study. Paraplegia. 1993;**31**:68-72

[44] Jankowski R, Zurkiel R, Nowak S, Czekanowska-Szlandrowicz R, Stachowska-Tomczak B. Vertebral column and spinal cord injuries: isolated and concomitant with multiple injury. Chiropractic Narzary Ruchun Ortopedia Policy. 1993;**58**:353-359

[45] Soopramanien A. Epidemiology of spinal injuries in Romania. Paraplegia. 1994;**32**:715-722

[46] Pedersen V, Muleer PG, Biering-Sorensen F. Traumatic spinal cord injuries in Groenland 1965-1986. Paraplegia. 1989;**27**:345-349

[47] Mazaira J, Labanda F, Romero J, García ME, Gambarruta C, Sánchez A, et al. Epidemiología de la lesión medular y otros aspectos. Rehabilitación (Madr). 1998;**32**:365-372

[48] García Reneses J, Herruzco Cabrera R, Martinez MM. Epidemiological study of spinal cord injury in Spain 1984-1985. Paraplegia. 1991;**28**:180-190

[49] García Reneses J, Herruzco CR. Epidemiología descriptiva de la prevalencia de la lesión medular en España. Médula Espinal. 1995;**1**:116-121

[50] García Bravo AM. Características epidemiológicas de la lesión medular traumática en la provincia de las Palmas. Apertura de la Unidad de Lesionados Medulares de Canarias y su impacto en la población afecta. Universidad de las Palmas de Gran Canarias, Gran Canarias. 2004

[51] García Bravo AM, Méndez Suárez JL, Bárbara Bataller E, Sánchez Enriquez J, Miranda Calderín G, Álvarez GC. Epidemiología de la lesión medular en la provincia de las Palmas. Rehabilitación (Madr). 2003;**37**:74-80

[52] Van den Berg M, Castellote JM, Mahillo-Fernández I, de Pedro CJ. Incidence of traumatic spinal cord injury in Aragon, Spain (1972-2008). Journal of Neurotrauma. 2011;**28**:469-477

[53] Alén Garabato JJ, López Navarro M, Ramírez GL, Castelló Verdú J, García DL. Epidemiología de la lesión medular por accidente de zambullida en el agua: revisión de 1974-1995. Médula Espinal. 1996;**3**:161-164

[54] Cripps R. Spinal cord injury, Australia, 2006-07. In: Injury Research and Statistics Series Number 48 Cat. No. INJCAT. Vol. 119. Adelaide: AIHW; 2008

[55] Dixon GS, Danesh JN, Caradoc-Davies TH. Epidemiology of spinal cord injury in New Zealand. Neuroepidemiology. 1993;**12**:88-95

[56] Maharaj JC. Epidemiology of spinal cord paralysis in Fiji: 1985-1994. Spinal Cord. 1996;**34**:549-559

[57] GBD. Global, regional, and national burden of traumatic brain injury and spinal cord injury, 1990-2016: a systematic analysis for the Global Burden of Disease Study 2016. Lancet Neurology. 2016;**2019**(18):56-87

[58] Price C, Makintubee S, Herndon W, Istre GR. Epidemiology of traumatic spinal cord injury and acute hospitalization and rehabilitation charges for spinal cord injuries in Oklahoma, 1988-1990. American Journal of Epidemiology. 1994;**139**:37-47

Chapter 2

Cauda Equina Syndrome

Mohammad Hanoun, Abdulnasser Thabet
and Abdullah Hanoun

Abstract

Cauda equina syndrome is a relatively rare clinical syndrome caused by compression of cauda equina and can result in significant morbidity if not treated. In this chapter, we describe briefly the anatomical background of the lumbar spine and the nerve supply of the urinary bladder, as the urinary symptoms play a crucial role in diagnosis of this syndrome. Then, we move on to discuss the etiology, symptoms, and signs of cauda equina syndrome. We also describe the different modalities to make the diagnosis including the CT scan, MRI, nerve conduction studies, and electromyogram. Finally, the management of this syndrome including the surgical procedures, complications, and prognosis. We enclosed five real-life cases of different causes of CES from our practice briefly describing the clinical background of the patients as well as CT and/ or MRI images of each case.

Keywords: CES: Cauda Equina Syndrome, CESI: Incomplete cauda equina syndrome, CESR: cauda equina syndrome retention, CNS: central nervous system, NCS: Nerve conduction studies, EMG: Electromyogram, MIS: Minimal Invasive Surgery, CSF: Cerebral Spinal Fluid

1. Introduction

Cauda equina syndrome (CES) is a relatively rare clinical condition caused by compression of the nerve roots forming the cauda equina (the tail end of the spinal cord). CES produces a characteristic set of clinical features and is a surgical emergency requiring urgent intervention to prevent permanent neurological deficits. In this chapter, we will discuss the anatomical background of the lumbar spine as well as clinical manifestations, causes, differential diagnosis, and management of this condition.

2. Anatomical background

Lumbar and sacral spine: Human body has five lumbar and five sacral vertebrae. Each vertebra consists of body and neural element which in turn composed of pedicles, laminae, spinous process, and two articular facets, namely superior and inferior.

An intervertebral disc is found between two successive vertebrae. The disc is formed by central nucleus pulposus and peripheral anulus fibrosis. The neural exit foramen is the space between two adjacent pedicles in the sagittal plane, and this space is normally filled with fat (**Figures 1–6**).

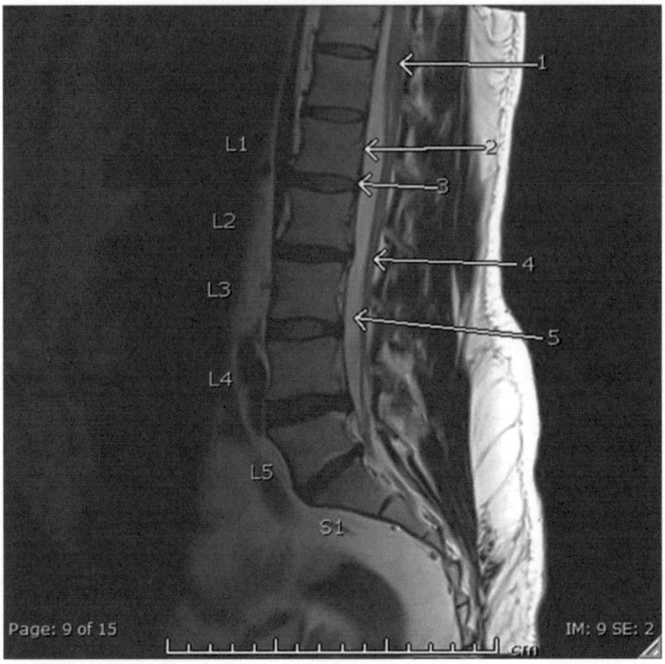

Figure 1.
1. Conus medullaris, 2. L1 vertebral body, 3. L1-L2 Intervertebral disc, 4. Cauda equina, 5. CSF within thecal sac.

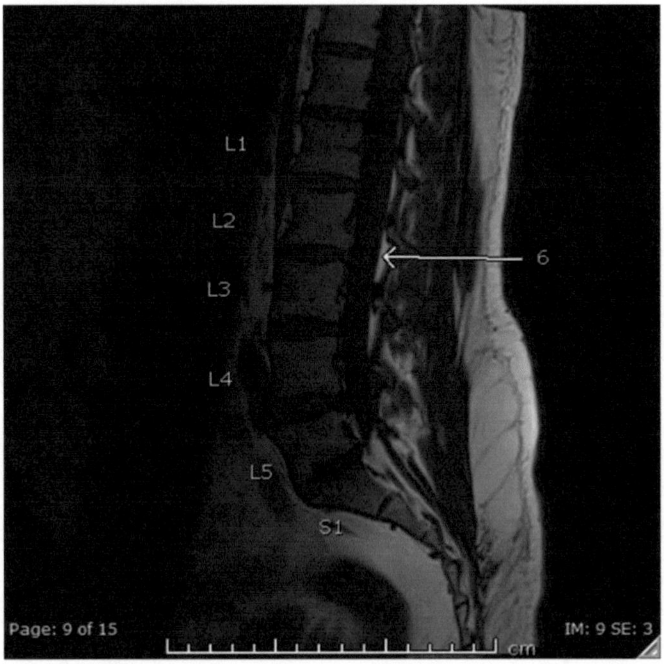

Figure 2.
6. Dorsal epidural fat.

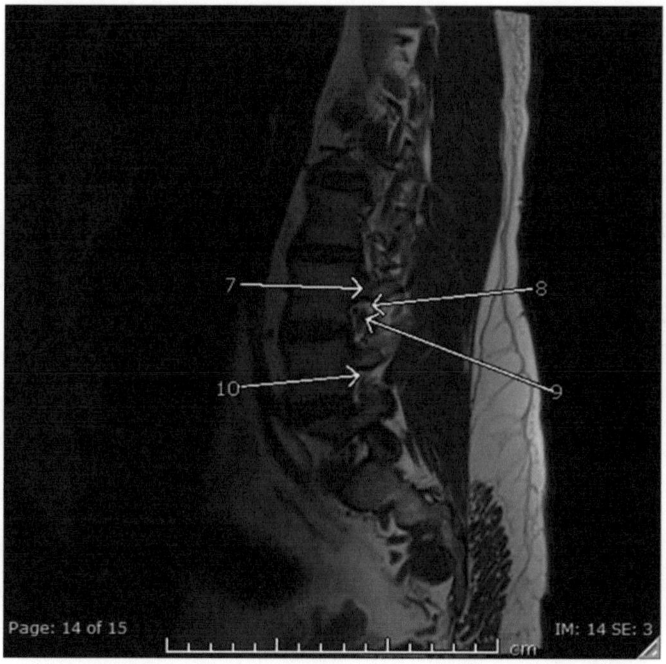

Figure 3.
7. Pedicle, 8. Fat within neural exit foramen, 9. Exiting nerve root, 10. Neural exit foramen.

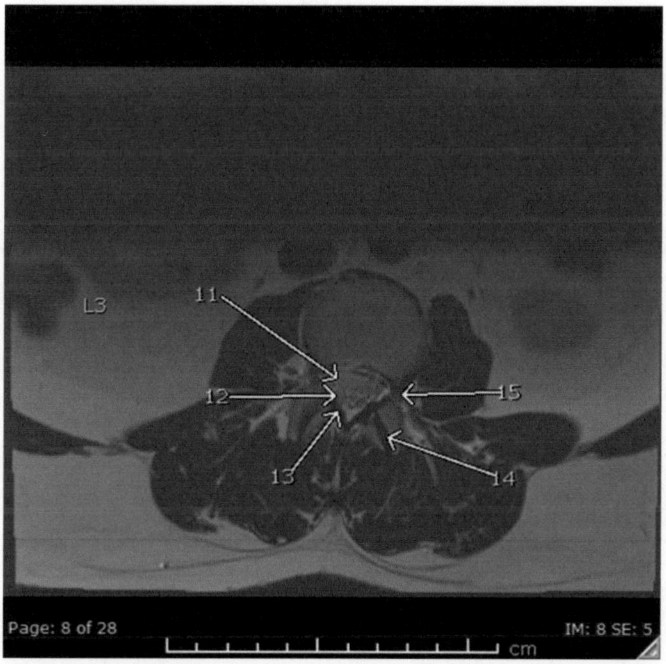

Figure 4.
11. CSF within thecal sac, 12. Cauda equina, 13. Ligamentum flavum, 14. Facet joint, 15. Pedicle.

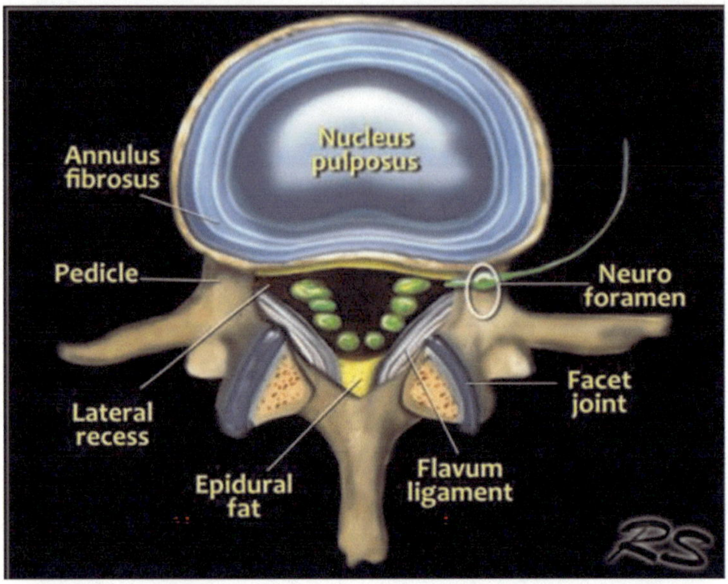

Figure 5.
Normal anatomy of lumbar vertebra with the neural elements and related structures.

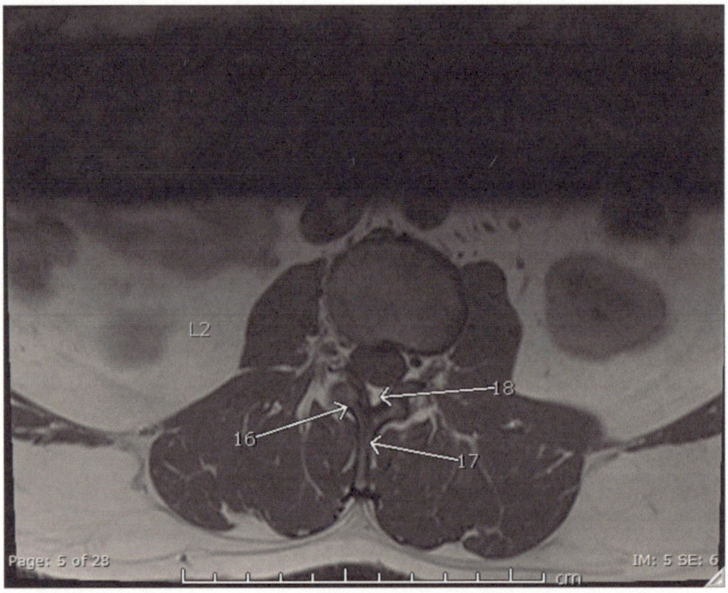

Figure 6.
16. Lamina, 17. Spinous process, 18. Dorsal epidural lipoma.

Spinal cord with the brain forms the central nervous system. The spinal cord starts at the cervicomedullary junction at the foramen magnum to the conus medullaris which is the terminal part of the cord, and this usually is seen at L1 level. Thirty-one pairs of nerve roots are seen arising from spinal cord as follows: 8 cervical, 12 thoracic, 5 lumbar, 5 sacral, and one coccygeal. In axial section, the spinal cord is formed of central gray and peripheral white matter.

Cauda equina: The name of cauda equina came from Latin language and means horse tail. Cauda equina is the collection of nerve roots within the thecal sac extending from conus medullaris to the sacral canal through the lumbar spine (**Figure 7**). As we go down two nerve roots, one on each side, leave thecal sac through the exit foramen which is located between the two successive pedicles in the sagittal plane, we call these nerves exiting nerves. At the same time, another nerve root (transiting nerve) on each side starts to go peripherally preparing itself to leave the thecal sac in the next level. Like a train, in each station, two passengers are leaving from doors on each side of the train, and at the same time, two passengers carry their baggage and start to approach the doors to prepare themselves to leave the train in the next station.

The exiting nerve roots of the lower lumbar (L4 and L5) and sacral (S1, S2, S3, and S4) spine interconnect together to form the lumbosacral plexus which serves motor and sensory functions to the pelvis and lower limbs. Pudendal nerve is a branch of the sacral plexus formed by S2–S4 sacral nerve roots. It plays an important role in urinary, anal, and sexual functions. It has three branches, namely:

- Perineal nerve: motor to muscles of the urogenital triangle and sensory to the perineal region.

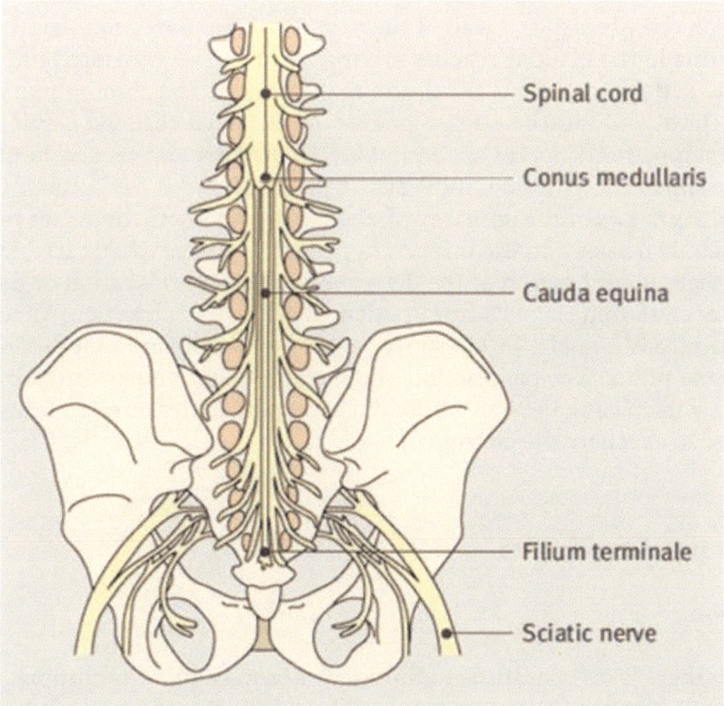

Figure 7.
Anatomy of the lumbosacral spine and the related cauda equina.

- Dorsal nerve of the penis (or clitoris): sensory.
- Inferior rectal nerve: motor to the external anal sphincter and sensory to perineal region.

The urinary symptoms are crucial in diagnosis and prognosis of the cauda equina syndrome as discussed later, and the nerve supply of the urinary bladder should be explained particularly.

The urinary bladder has normally autonomic and sensory blood supply as follows;

- Autonomic nerve supply:

  Sympathetic supply from L1 and L2. The effect of this type inhibits the contraction of the detrusor muscle which forms the wall of the urinary bladder and compress the internal urethral sphincter to prevent micturition.

  Parasympathetic supply from S1, S2, S3, and S4. The parasympathetic supply antagonizes the sympathetic effect leading to contraction of the muscle and relaxation of the sphincter.

- Sensory nerve fibers from the urinary bladder to spinal cord [1].

3. Micturition reflex

The stretch receptors in the wall of the urinary bladder are stimulated when the volume of urine in the bladder reaches around 300 ml. The generated impulses reach CNS, and the body starts to feel the desire to pass urine. The coming impulses reach the second, third, and fourth sacral segments of the spinal cord via pelvic splanchnic nerves. The sympathetic nerves send impulses to the first and second lumbar segments of the spinal cord through hypogastric plexuses. From the second, third, and fourth sacral segments of the spinal cord, the parasympathetic impulses pass through pelvic splanchnic nerves and the inferior hypogastric plexus to urinary bladder wall. As a result, there is contraction of the detrusor muscle and relaxation of the sphincter, which also receives some signals from pudendal nerve for relaxation. When the urine reaches urethra, additional afferent signals from the urethra are sent to the spinal cord to reinforce the reflex. The contraction of the abdominal muscles can also help in micturition by increasing the intraabdominal and pelvic pressures and therefore compress bladder to evacuate the contents [1].

4. Cauda equina syndrome

4.1 Definition

Although there is no consensus definition for cauda equina syndrome, this lower motor neuron condition occurs when there is dysfunction of cauda equina, precisely S2 and below nerve roots [2]. This usually occurs due to mechanical compression.

4.2 Epidemiology

It is considered a rare entity with a prevalence estimated by approximately 1 in 65,000 in one study [3]. It is seen in around 3% of lumbar spine disc herniation.

4.3 Etiology

Cauda equina syndrome occurs when there is significant spinal canal stenosis and mechanical compression on cauda equina enough to produce symptoms. The commonest cause is disc herniation. Other less common causes are neoplasms, trauma, hematoma, abscess, and inflammation (**Table 1**) [3].

4.4 Disc disease

This is the commonest cause for spinal canal stenosis and cauda equina syndrome [2–5]. Disc herniation is displacement of disc material like nucleus pulposus, parts of the annulus fibrosus, and cartilage, beyond the limits of the intervertebral disc space (**Figure 8**). This can be either diffuse (disc bulge) or focal (herniation). Focal disc herniation can be further subdivided into protrusion (broad base at parent disc), extrusion (narrow or no base at parent disc), and extrusion with sequestration (extruded disc without contiguity to parent disc) [6], (see Case 1).

MRI shows disc extrusion at L4-L5 compressing cauda equina.

Had surgical laminectomy and microdiscectomy, 2 months after surgery patient still complains of weakness in the lower limbs with urinary incontinence and constipation (**Figures 9** and **10**).

The central spinal canal stenosis and cauda equina compression by degenerative disc disease are commonly associated by other risk factors like hypertrophic facet joint arthropathy and ligamentum flavum thickening as well as spondylolisthesis [6] and epidural lipomatosis [7, 8].

Disc herniation
Trauma
Spinal stenosis
Tumors: primary and secondary
Infection
Arteriovenous malformation
Hemorrhage (subarachnoid, subdural, epidural)
Ankylosing spondylitis
Iatrogenic causes
Continuous spinal anesthesia
Postsurgery
Postintradiscal therapy
Postchiropractic manipulation

Table 1.
Causes of Cauda Equina syndrome.

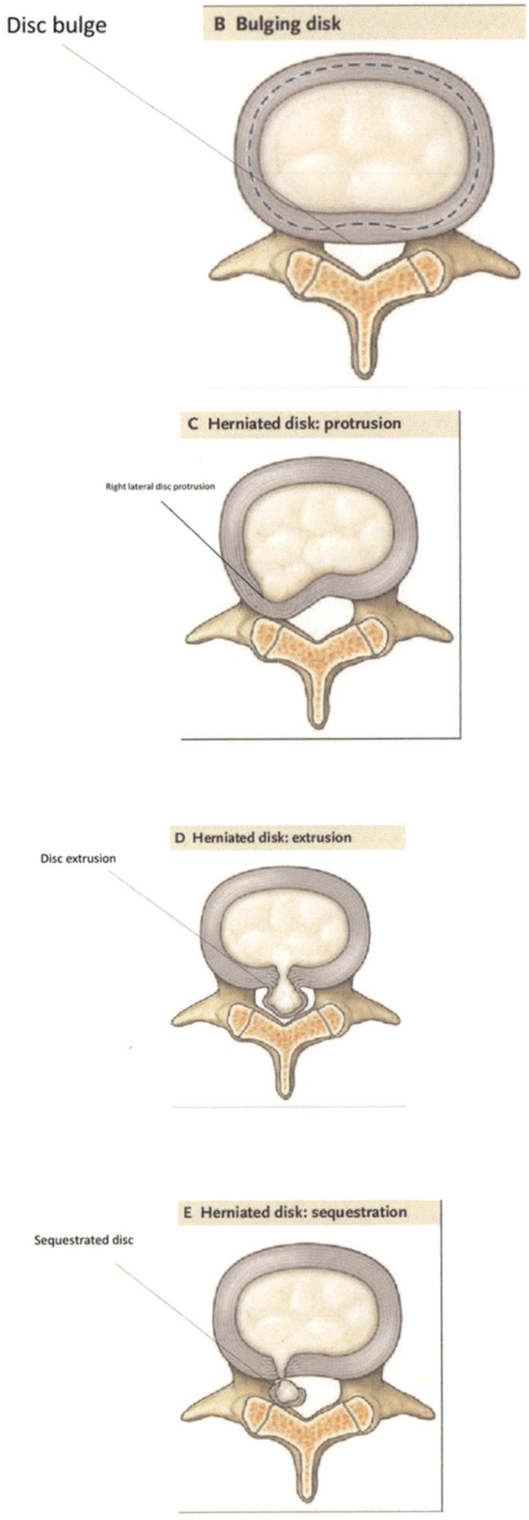

Figure 8.
Classification of degenerative disc disease.

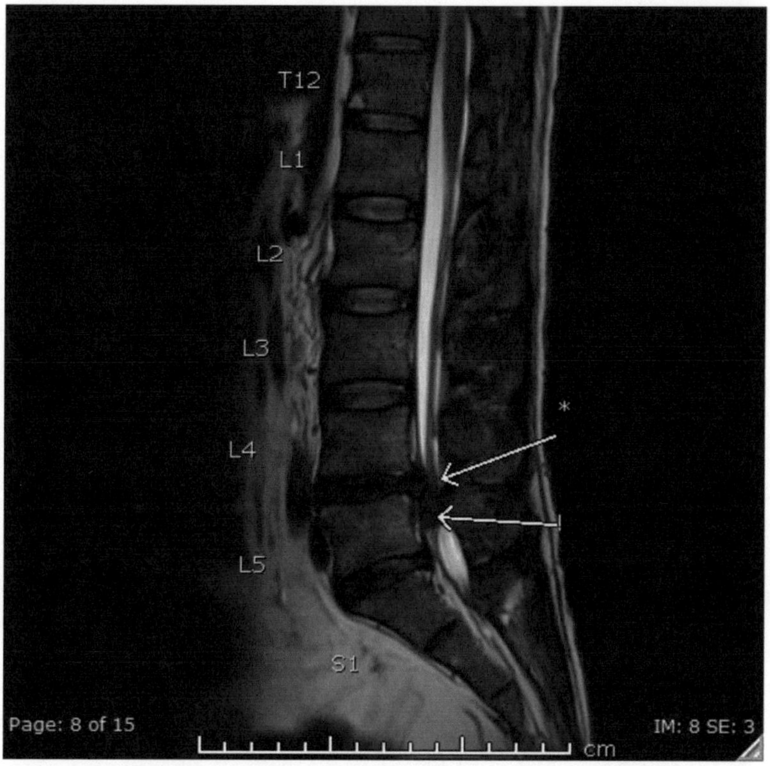

Figure 9.
Sagittal T2 showing disc extrusion (!), compressed cauda equina (*).

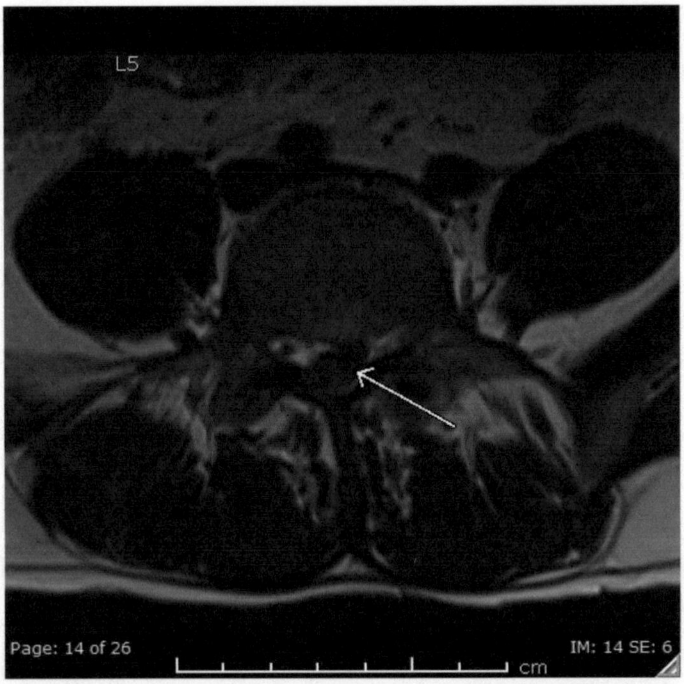

(a)

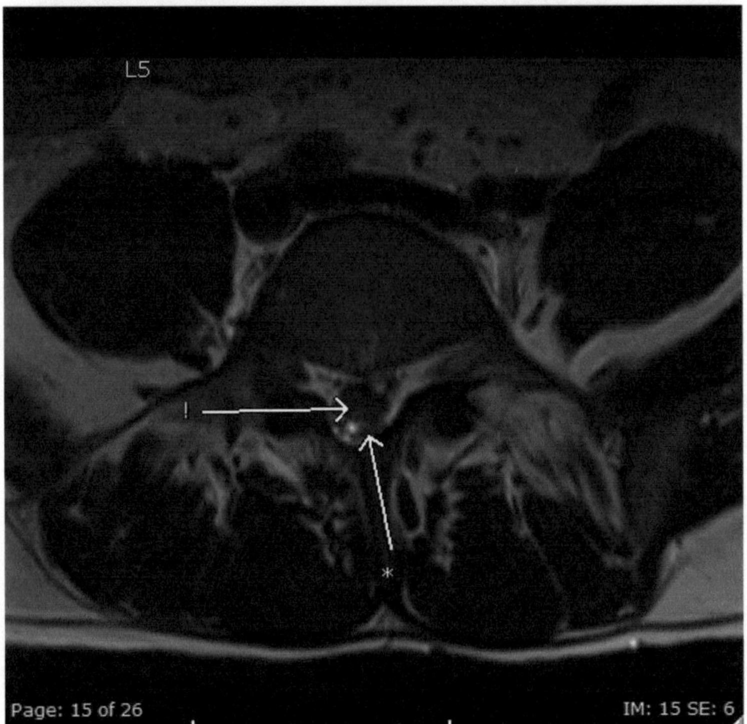

(b)

Figure 10.
Axial T2 showing extruded disc (!), compressed cauda equina (*).

4.5 Neoplasms

Primary:

- Myxopapillary ependymoma: intradural extramedullary tumor arises from ependymal glia of the filum terminale. It is usually seen below conus medullaris [9].
- Schwannoma: benign intradural extramedullary tumor. It is the commonest nerve sheath tumor of the spine (**Figure 11**).
- Meningioma: intradural extramedullary spinal canal tumor arises from spinal meninges. It is more common in female [3].

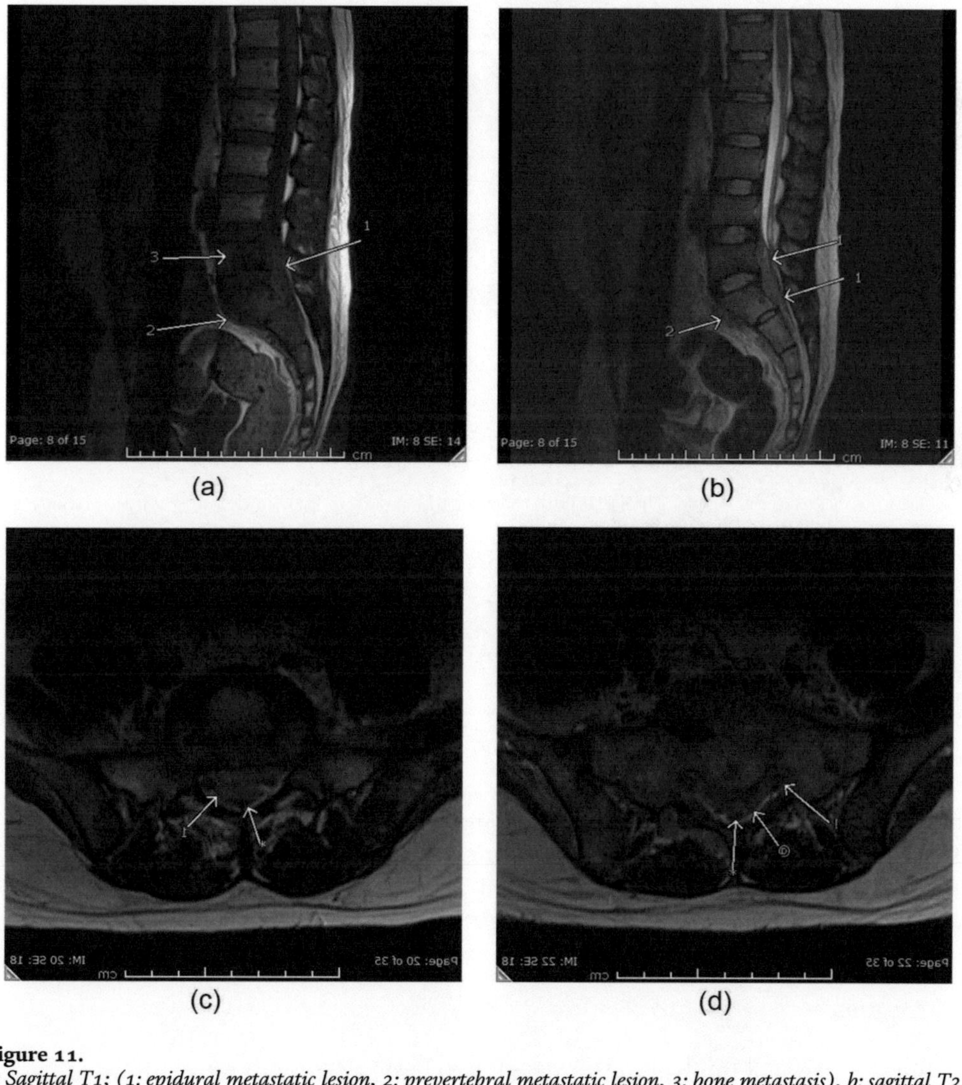

Figure 11.
*a: Sagittal T1; (1: epidural metastatic lesion, 2: prevertebral metastatic lesion, 3: bone metastasis), b: sagittal T2; (1: epidural metastatic lesion, 2: prevertebral metastatic lesion), c and b: axial T2; (1: epidural metastatic lesion, *: cauda equina, !: S1 exiting nerve root, @: S2 transiting nerve root).*

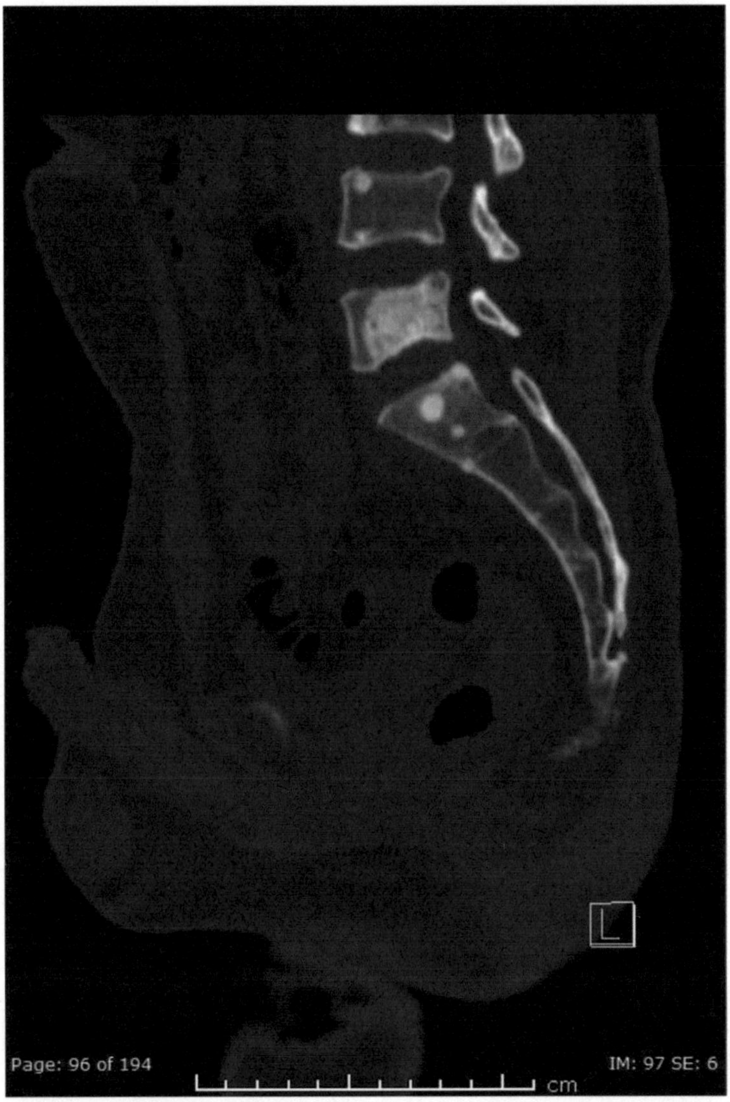

Figure 12.
CT scan showing multiple sclerotic bone metastasis.

Secondary (metastasis): can be either from CNS through drop metastasis (where the primary tumors usually high grade glioma, germinoma, medulloblastoma, and choroid plexus tumors), or hematogenous metastasis from outside the CNS commonly lung and breast primaries [4, 10]. Metastasis can be from outside CNS commonly lung and breast malignancies (see Case 2) (**Figures 12** and **13**).

4.6 Trauma

Burst fracture of lumbar and/or sacral vertebral bodies with retropulsion of fractured fragments or vertebral subluxation may encroach on the spinal canal and compress cauda equina causing this syndrome (see Case 3) (**Figures 14** and **15**).

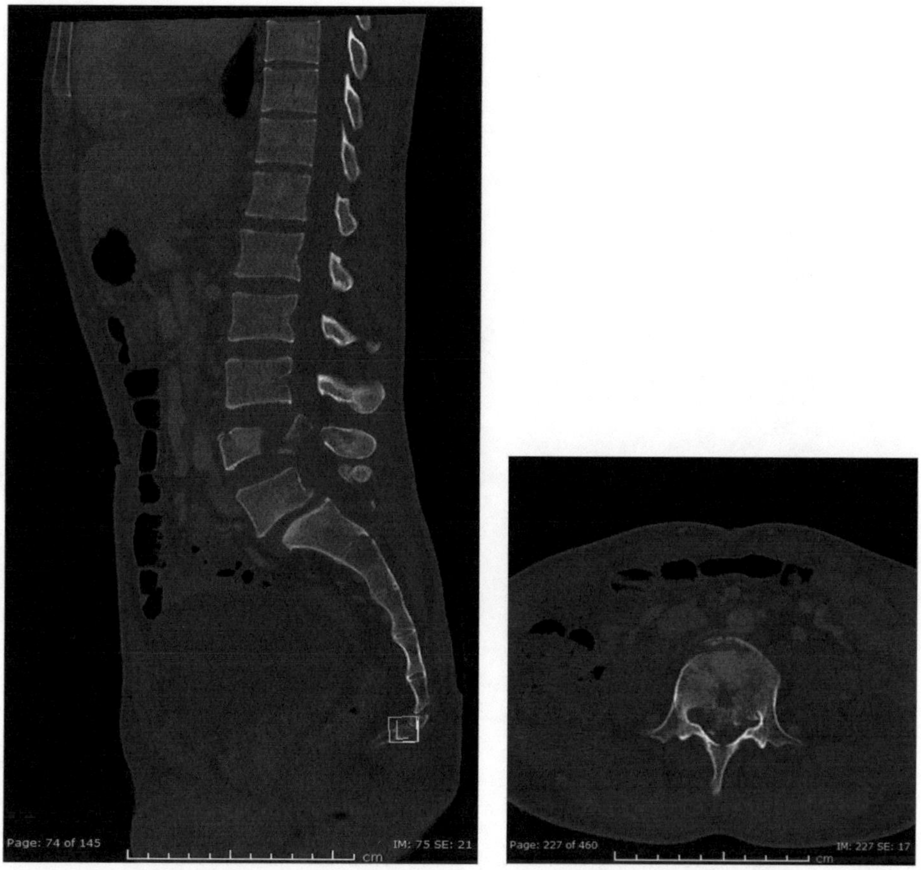

(a) (b)

Figure 13.
Burst fracture of L4 vertebral body with retropulsion encroaching on the spinal canal.

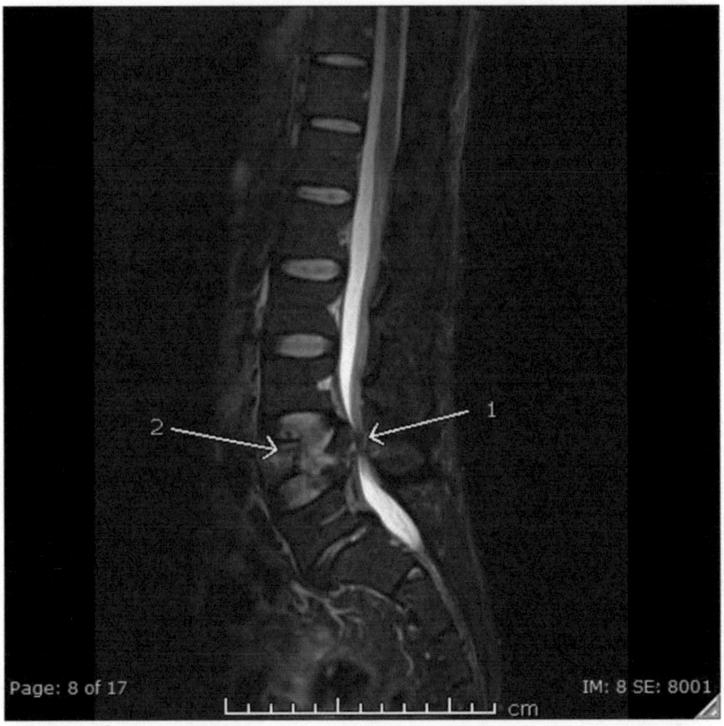

(a)

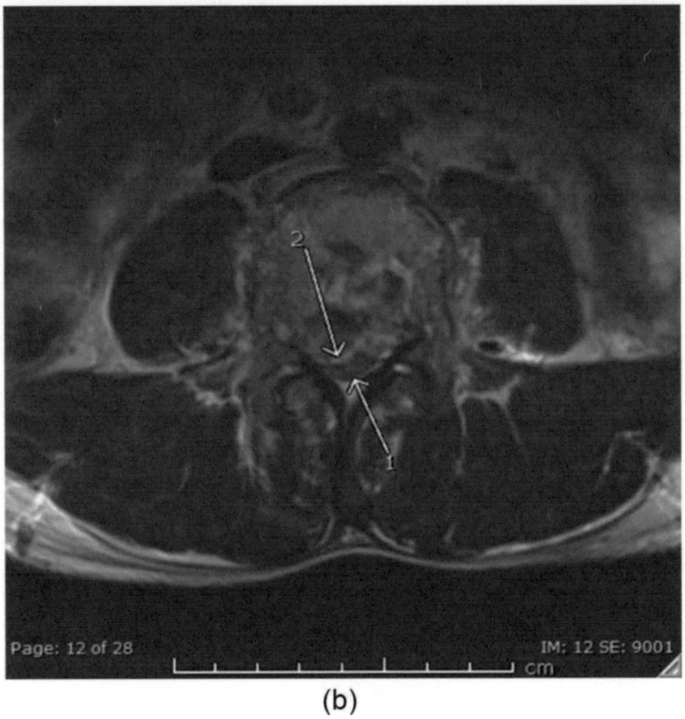

(b)

Figure 14.
(a) Sagittal STIR showing 1: compressed cauda equina, 2: fractured vertebral body (b) Axial T2 showing compressed cauda equina 1 and the fractured vertebral body.

This can be also sometimes associated with significant hematoma adding to cauda equina compression and spinal canal stenosis.

4.7 Infection

- Tuberculous spondylodiscitis: Inflamed soft tissue (phlegmon) with abscess can compress the cauda equina and cause significant spinal canal stenosis.
- Pyogenic spondylitis: Sizable pyogenic abscess can compress cauda equina and produce symptoms (see Case 4).

MRI Exam showed anterior epidural collection along the lumbar spine compressing cauda equina. It also showed enhancement of L5 and S1 vertebral body suggesting spondylitis. Surgical drainage of spinal abscess was done. There was significant improvement with almost complete recovery after surgical drainage and full course of bacterial antibiotics (**Figure 15**).

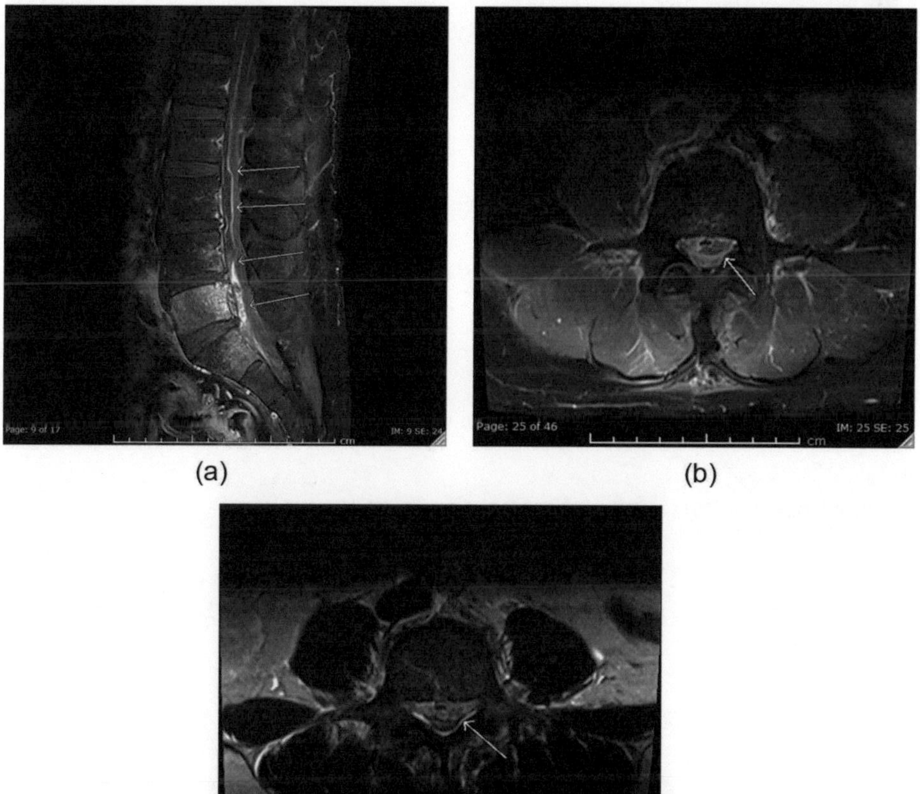

Figure 15.
a: Sagittal T1 post contrast and b: axial T1 post contrast: shows epidural collection with marginal enhancement. c: axial T2: shows bright collection compressing cauda equina.

4.8 Inflammatory

A rare cause of CES is ankylosing spondylitis [11, 12]: This is a chronic progressive inflammatory disease of the joints which can cause ligamentous calcification and osteophyte formation, and this may result in significant spinal canal stenosis and cauda equina compression.

4.9 Degenerative

Synovial cysts, spondylolisthesis, facet joint arthropathy, and hypertrophy of ligamentum flavum can cause canal stenosis; however, these more commonly add to spinal canal stenosis in the presence of other factors like disc herniation (**Figure 16**) [3, 13, 14].

Hematoma: can be due to trauma, bleeding tendency, or iatrogenic this can be a cause.

Epidural lipomatosis: This can rarely alone cause CES [15]. This is usually related to prolonged use of corticosterioids, obesity, or idiopathic [16].

4.10 Symptoms and signs

Symptoms depend grossly on the degree of compression and the nerve roots being compressed.

The following are the symptoms seen in cauda equina syndrome:

1. Lower back pain.

2. Unilateral or bilateral leg pain (sciatica). *Bilateral sciatica should be always taken seriously.*

3. Unilateral or bilateral lower limb weakness.

4. Saddle anesthesia: This includes perineal and perianal areas as well as inner thighs, and the severity of the sensory disturbance correlates with the number of the involved nerve roots.

5. Bladder, bowl or sexual dysfunction; the later two are only rarely seen.

Although all these symptoms can be seen in cauda equina syndrome, the latter two [4 and 5] are the hallmarks for definite diagnosis [2, 3].

4.11 Presentation

The onset of symptoms can be either acute (rare), acute on top of chronic (commonest presentation) or chronic [2].

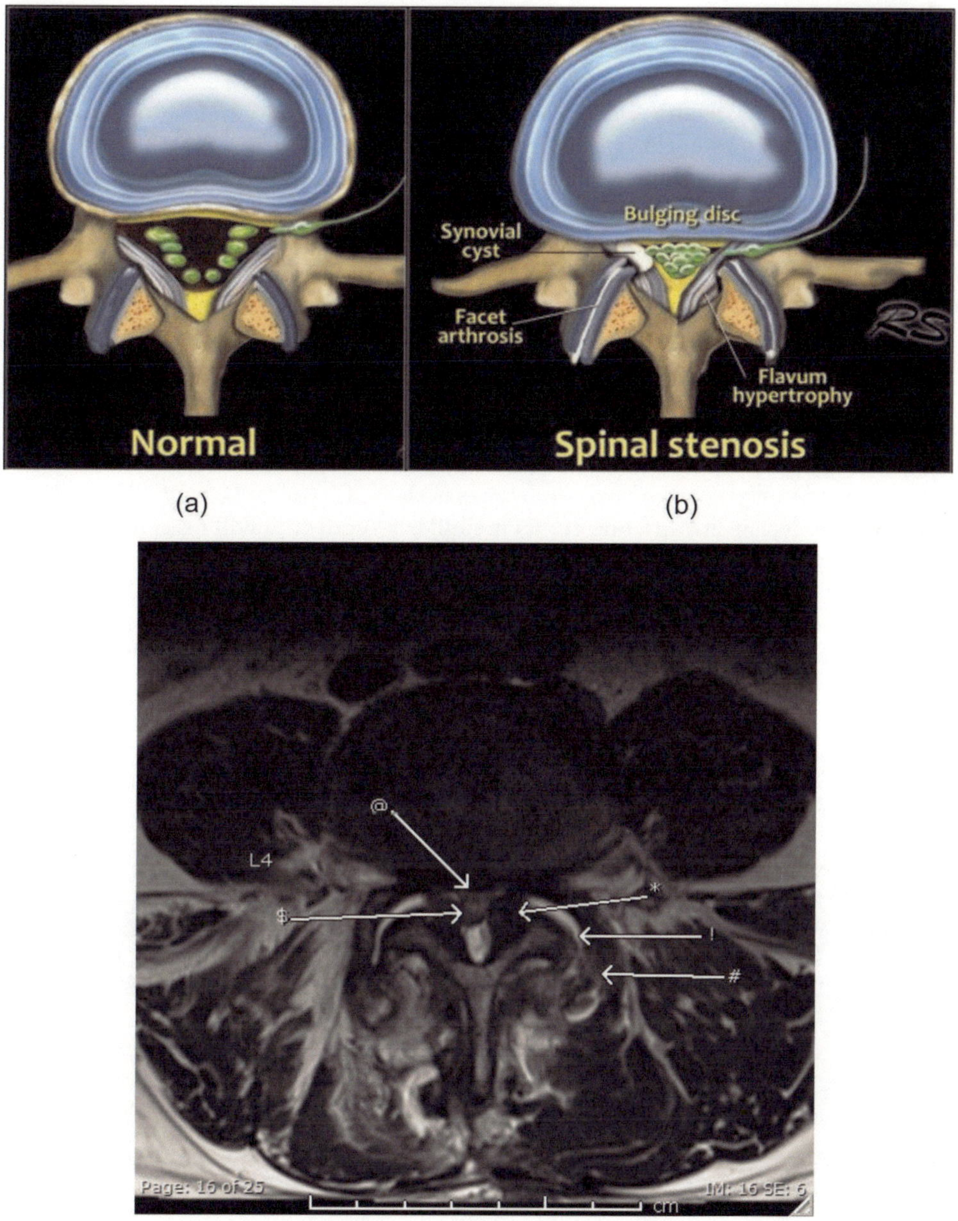

Figure 16.
*@: Protruding disc, $: Compressed cauda equina within thecal sac, *: Thickened ligamentum flavum, !: Joint effusion, #: Hypertrophied facet joint.*

4.12 Classification of CES

This widely used classification to assess the severity of the damage and predict the outcome of CES was proposed by **Gleave and Macfarlane**, and accordingly CES is classified to incomplete CES (CESI) and CES with painless bladder retention/ CES (CESR).

In CESI, the patient has urinary difficulties of neurogenic origin such as altered urinary sensation, loss of desire to void, poor stream or the need to strain, but there is still executive control of bladder function and voiding is possible even if difficult.

Meanwhile CESR occurs when the bladder is no longer under executive control and there is painless retention of urine with overflow [2, 5].

Another less commonly used classification was proposed by J Shi and et al. based on the clinical presentation and physiological disability, where CES is classified into four stages, namely preclinical, early, middle, and late. However, this classification has not been widely adopted by the neurosurgeons community [17].

4.13 Differential diagnosis

The main differential diagnosis is conus medullaris syndrome (see Case 5), the main difference between the two syndromes is that CES presents only with lower motor neuron deficit, meanwhile conus medullaris syndrome will present with signs of both upper and lower motor neuron lesion.

MRI with IV contrast was done. It showed extramedullary lesion at T12-L1 level compressing conus medullaris (**Figure 17**). This was surgically resected. In histopathological examination the lesion was proved to be schwannoma. Patient showed significant improvement after surgical resection.

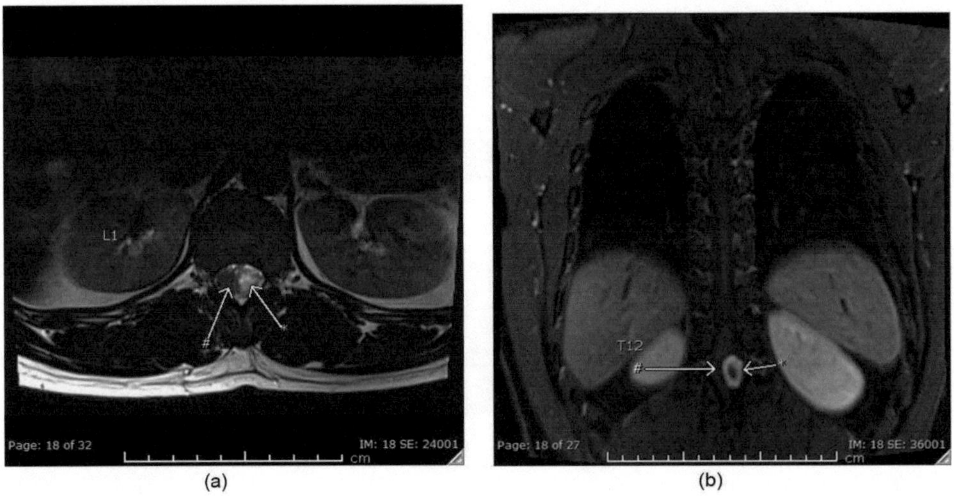

Figure 17.
**: Lesion, #: Conus medullaris.*

4.14 Investigation

Cauda equina syndrome is a clinical condition. Imaging plays an important role in detecting the cause of this condition. MRI is the best modality and is enough in most patients. In case of CES, MRI will reveal the cause in most of the patients, which can be large disc herniation, tumor, or collection (which can be either hematoma or abscess) compressing cauda equina nerve roots. There will be usually significant spinal canal stenosis. From the radiological point of view, central spinal canal stenosis of the lumbar spine can be classified based on the cauda equina nerve root aggregation. Grade 1 (mild stenosis) is when the anterior CSF space is mildly obliterated, but all the nerves in the cauda equina can be clearly separated from each other. Grade 2 or moderate stenosis indicates cauda equina aggregation, while grade 3 signifies severe stenosis with the entire cauda equina appearing as a one bundle (**Figures 18** and **19**) [6].

CT is a good alternative when the MRI is contra indicated, and it is very good in assessing bony tissues and bony spinal canal stenosis. CT scan can highly exclude cauda equina impingement if the thecal sac is effaced by less than 50%, as one study concluded [18]. The possibility of CT to identify soft tissue lesions can be sometimes limited by artifacts. Myelogram is another modality; however, it is considered relatively invasive as it requires intrathecal injection of contrast.

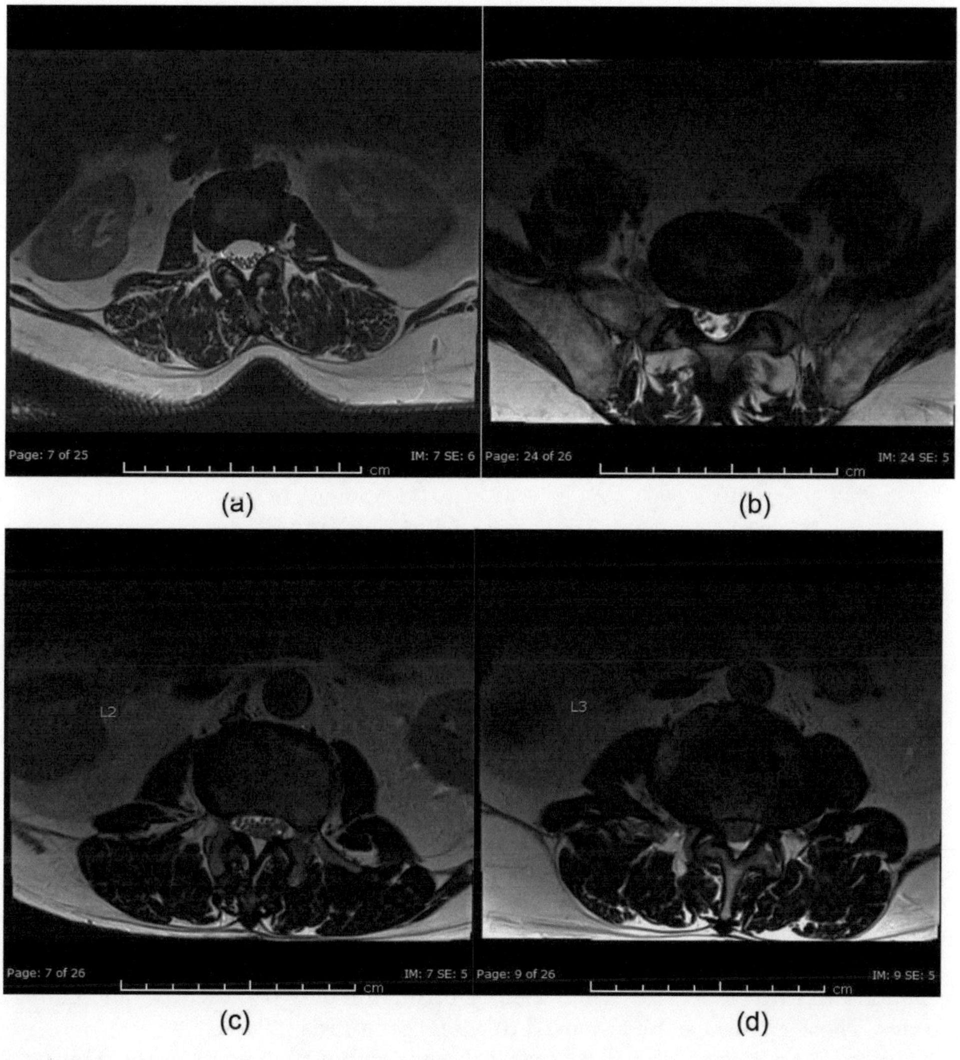

Figure 18.
Degrees of central spinal canal stenosis: (a) no stenosis (b) mild canal stenosis (c) mild canal stenosis (d) severe canal stenosis.

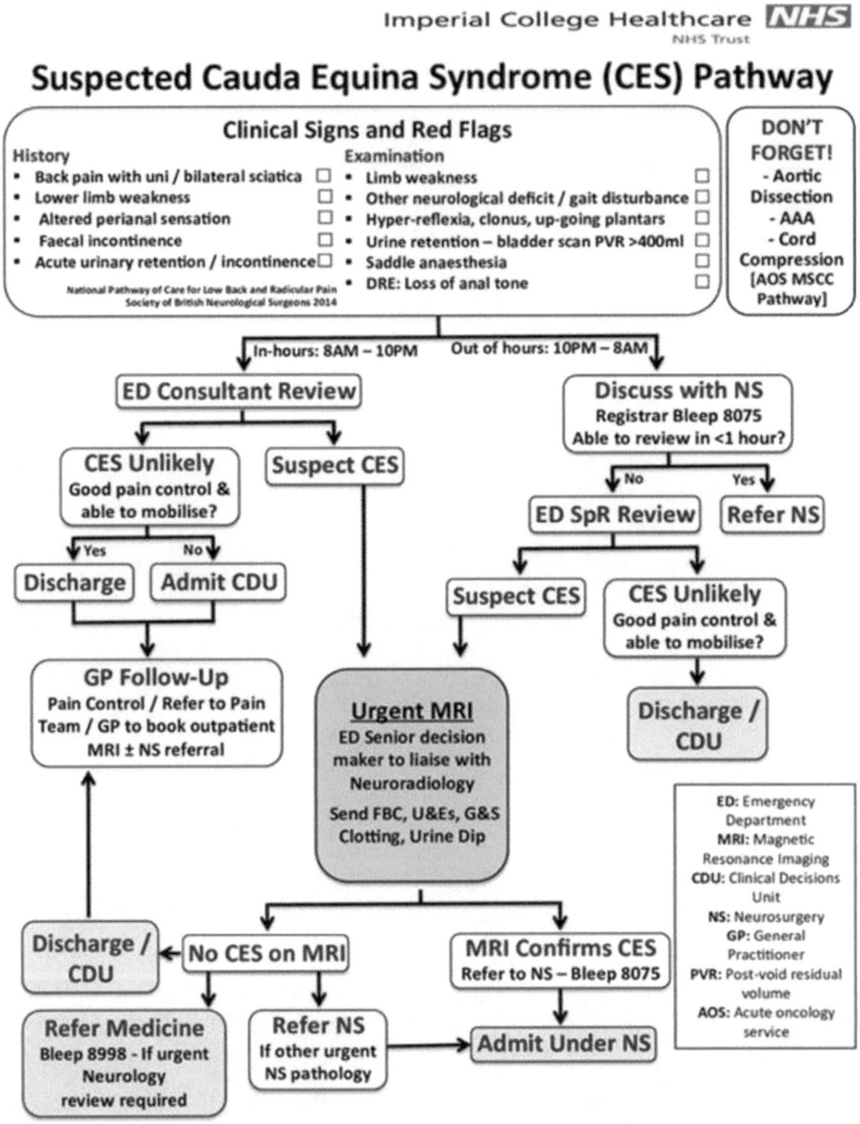

Figure 19.
Summary of the management pathway for suspected cauda equina syndrome cases in the Charing Cross Hospital (CXH) ED. NHS, National Health Service UK.

Nerve conduction studies (NCS) and electromyogram (EMG): These are two electrodiagnostic tests frequently done together to assess the functional integrity of the targeted nerve and therefore the degree and extent of nerve damage (which cannot be achieved by imaging). When done together, they have high specificity and sensitivity regarding the involved nerve root. Electrodiagnostic tests are usually complementary to MRI, especially when there is mismatch between the MRI and clinical findings. These exams can be also used to assess prognosis [19].

They are more helpful in patients with chronic rather than acute onset. This is because abnormality in EMG needs at least two weeks from the clinical onset to be detected (**Figure 19**) [10].

4.15 Treatment

Indications of surgery:
Absolute indications to the surgical decompression include.

- Compressive etiologies.
- Acute to subacute progression of neurologic deficits including lower limb weakness and bladder disturbances.

The surgical intervention is the only option for preventing further deterioration and for recovery, either open microdiscectomy or MIS.

Surgical issue: Some advise a bilateral laminectomy (but this is not mandatory).

Time of surgery: Most evidence supports within 24 hours is desirable if possible, some evidence supports that surgery within 48 is acceptable, and after that the chance of recovery is less and less. The Standard surgery is open microscopic lumbar laminotomy/ laminectomy and discectomy [20] microdiscectomy similar to standard procedure, but a smaller incision is utilized.

Advantages may be cosmetic, shortened hospital stay, and lower blood loss. Overall efficacy is similar to standard discectomy.

4.16 Steps of the procedure

Great care should be taken to position the patient correctly on the operating table to avoid pressure sores and neural peripheral nerve compression. As known, excessive abdominal compression during the prone position can result in excessive epidural bleed due to venous congestion. Landmarks for skin incision are the spinous processes, posterior superior iliac spine, and iliac wings.

A line that is drawn between the posterior superior iliac spines usually projects to the disk level of L4–15. However, this is unreliable, and image intensifier control is necessary in every case.

For CES secondary to lumbar stenosis, the principal surgical option is decompression +/− fusion.

The aim of decompression is to create more room for nerves and thecal sac and release the compression from soft tissue structures as the following disk herniation, hypertrophic ligamentum flavum, hypertrophic facet joints, osteophytes, and narrowed bony canal [21].

Performing complete laminectomies in the past was the standard method for decompression in central spinal stenosis. But from other hand found that complete laminectomies may increase chances of instability at those levels. Recently inter-laminar approaches involve leaving intact portions of the lamina and the connection between the facet joints, laminae, and pedicles, and pars interarticularis approach significantly reduces the chance of instability.

A midline approach exposes the inter-laminar windows at L3–L4 and L4–L5 as well as the facet joints to decompress a spinal stenosis at these levels.

The decompression inter-lamina is opened with a Kerrison rongeur half of laminae, ligamentum flavum, and hypertrophy facet. It is important to release that the narrowest part of the stenosis is typically under the lamina. The remaining part needs to be undercut from the superior and inferior sides, respectively. In some cases, decompression and fusion are necessary where the spine is deemed unstable. In the case of tumor or inflammation, decompressive laminectomies alone are rarely indicated. The goals of surgical intervention are better accomplished by combining decompression of neural structures, debulking of tumor mass, realignment of spinal deformity, and spinal reconstruction with instrumentation and bone grafting.

4.17 Post-operative actions

Several therapeutic options are available for patients with CES post operation, according to its underlying cause.

- Anti-inflammatory agents including corticosteroids (especially methylprednisolone) can be effective in patients with inflammatory processes, including ankylosing spondylitis.

- Patients with CES caused by an infection should receive appropriate antibiotic therapy.

- Patients affected by CE neoplasms confirmed by tissue [22].

Sampling should be evaluated for chemotherapy and radiation therapy.

- In most cases, treatment with medications alone is not indicated because of a need for emergency release of nerve compression.

- If CES is due to tumors, traumas, metabolic diseases (i.e., lipomatosis), or chronic inflammation, a staged surgery with initial decompression and subsequent operation to correct the underlying cause may be the best approach. This can provide the greatest chance of resolution of CES, without compromising the treatment of the underlying pathology [23].

4.18 Contraindications

- Patients not suitable for surgery due to significant comorbidities or advanced age.

4.19 Complications

Complications can be classified into two groups:

- Procedure-specific complications (i.e., problems related to surgical approach or spinal implants)

- General postsurgical complications (may involve the neuro-logic, pulmonary, cardiovascular, and gastrointestinal systems).

Potential causes of neurologic deficits diagnosed after spine procedures include

- Direct intraoperative trauma to neural structures

- Acute vascular etiologies (including intraoperative hypotension, disruption of crucial segmental vessels supplying the spinal cord during anterior surgical approaches)

- Patient malpositioning during surgery (including brachial plexus injuries, compressive neuropathy involving the peroneal nerve)
- Post-operative bleeding with resultant epidural hematoma and neuronal compression
- Persistent pain
- Bone graft migration with resultant neurologic compromise
- Deep venous thrombosis (DVT)
- Instrumentation failure and/or persistent instability (e.g., due to nonunion or pseudoarthrosis).

4.20 Outcomes and prognosis

The prognosis for CES has traditionally been determined by multiple factors including

- Etiology
- Speed of onset and progression of symptoms: It seems that a more rapid onset corresponds to a poorer outcome
- Duration of compression: Immediate surgical decompression is often recommended to minimize the chances of permanent nerve injury
- Degree of neurologic deficit [20]
- Symptoms and signs: Bladder and/or anal sphincter disturbances or perianal anesthesia seems to be correlated with poor prognosis
- Levels of spinal involvement

5. Rehabilitation program

CES is one of the most common pathology post-surgeries need extensive rehabilitation programs. It is an emergency and needs to be managed by a multidisciplinary team. Rehabilitation programs are the most important part of multidisciplinary team after surgery of CES [24].

A proper rehabilitation results in making the patient functionally able in performing activities of daily living with ease.

Following 4–6 weeks of rehabilitation given significant improvement in movement, muscle strength, pain reduction, and functional sphincters.

6. Conclusions of CES

- CES is a complex of symptoms, and signs need urgent intervention.

- The surgery interventions are a mandatory option for CES to save lower limbs and sphincter function.
- Early intervention within 48 hours from onset will be good results.
- Delay intervention, the lower-extremity motor weakness that occasionally progresses to paraplegia or not improvement after surgery.
- Patients with CES should have undergone rapid radiologic evaluation and diagnosis.
- Lumbosacral trauma: It is important to maintain a high index of suspicion for the diagnosis of CES and its implications both diagnostically and prognostically.
- If the clinician has suspicious, this is a cauda equina syndrome,should obtain a post-void residual urine volume. In addition, trauma patients often receive an indwelling catheter at the time of admission to the emergency department.
- A rectal examination and evaluation of perianal sensation is mandatory when assessing any patient with acute onset of severe back pain or significant lumbosacral trauma.
- If an MRI is inadequate or contraindications, a CT-myelography) is alternative.
- For good results the rehabilitation after surgery is the key point for recovery or improvement.

7. Case reports of Cauda equina syndrome

- **Case 1:** 39 year old male patient complaining of more than one year history of back pain, presented to ED complaining of tingling sensation in the pelvis and thighs, with acute urinary retention since one day.
- **Case 2:** 34 year old patient with lung cancer with 2 weeks history of back pain, presented to ED complaining of new onset of saddle anesthesia ,urinary and stool incontinence. Physical exam shows lower limb weakness (**Figures 12** and **13**).
- **Case 3:** 35 year old male patient sustained multiple fractures after full from height complaining of severe back pain and urinary retention. CT Showed burst fracture of L4 vertebral body encroaching on the spinal canal. MRI revealed compression of cauda equina by the displaced bone fragment (**Figures 14** and **15**).
- **Case 4:** 50-year-old diabetic and hypertensive male patient presented to ED complaining of acute back pain and lower limb weakness with urine retention and perianal paresthesia. Patient was febrile. Blood test showed significant leukocytosis.
- **Case 5:** 38 year old male patient presented with progressive right sciatica, decreased sensation over the right lower limb as well as urine and stool incontinence of the last one month. Deep tendon reflexes were increased in physical examination. Diagnosed as conus medullaris syndrome.

DOI: http://dx.doi.org/10.5772/intechopen.109722

Conflict of interest

No conflict of interest.

Author details

Mohammad Hanoun[1]*, Abdulnasser Thabet[2] and Abdullah Hanoun[3]

1 Consultant Neuroradiologist, Neuroscience Institute, Hamad Medical Corporation, Doha, Qatar

2 Consultant Neurosurgeon, Neuroscience Institute, Hamad Medical Corporation, Doha, Qatar

3 FRCS, Manchester, UK

*Address all correspondence to: mhanoun@hamad.qa

References

[1] Richard SS et al. Clinical Anatomy by Regions. 8th ed. Philadelphia, USA: Lippincott Williams & Wilkins

[2] Lavy C, Marks P, Dangas K, Todd N. Cauda equina syndrome—A practical guide to definition and classification. International Orthopaedics. 2022; **46**(2):165-169. Published online 2021 Dec 4. DOI: 10.1007/s00264-021-05273-1

[3] Forsthoefel C, Moore DW. Cauda Equina Syndrome – Spine – Orthobulle ts, spine/2065/7/30/2021

[4] McNamee J, Flynn P, O'Leary S, Love M, Kelly B. Imaging in cauda Equina syndrome – A pictorial review. The Ulster Medical Journal. 2013;**82**(2): 100-108

[5] Gardner A, Gardner E, Morley T. Cauda equina syndrome: A review of the current clinical and medico-legal position. European Spine Journal. 2011; **20**(5):690-697. Published online 2010 Dec 31. DOI: 10.1007/s00586-010-1668-3

[6] Sergiy V, Glushko T, Jarraya M, Schuleri KH, Preul MC, Brooks ML, et al. ABCs of the degenerative spine. Insights Imaging. 2018;**9**(2):253-274. DOI: 10.1007/s13244-017-0584-z

[7] Knipe H. Spinal stenosis, Spinal ste nosis | Radiology Reference Article | Rad iopaedia.org, 2023

[8] Hadidi O, Hijazi H, Pajda R, Thomas B. Spinal epidural lipomatosis and focal Posterior longitudinal ligament hypertrophy causing severe cauda equina crowding. BMJ. 2022 Sep 30; **15**(9):e250112. DOI: 10.1136/bcr-2022-250112

[9] Yap J. Myxopapillary ependymoma | Radiology Reference Article | Radiopaed ia.org, 2022

[10] Hur JW, Park D-H, Lee J-B, Cho T-H, Park J-Y. Guidelines for Cauda Equina Syndrome Management, Department of Neurosurgery, College of Medicine, Korea University, Seoul, Korea. Journal of Neurointensive Care. 2019;**2**(1):14-16. DOI: 10.32587/jnic.2019.00136

[11] Tang C, Moser FG, Reveille J, et al. Cauda Equina syndrome in Ankylosing Spondylitis: Challenges in diagnosis, management, and pathogenesis. 2019; **46**(12):1582-1588. DOI: 10.3899/jrheum.181259

[12] Dakwar E, Reddy J, Vale FL, Uribe JS. A review of the pathogenesis of ankylosing spondylitis. Neurosurgery Focus. 2008;**24**(1):E2. DOI: 10.3171/FOC/2008/24/1/E2

[13] Shaw M, Birch N. Facet joint cysts causing cauda equina compression. 10.1097/01.bsd.0000112086.85112.cf

[14] Vadera S. Ligamentum flavum hype rtrophy | Radiology Reference Article | Radiopaedia.org, 2021

[15] Bushkar JB, Menkinsmith LP, Krywko DM. Idiopathic spinal epidural lipomatosis causing cauda Equina syndrome. Clinical Practice Cases Emerging Medicine. 2017;**1**(4):305-308. DOI: 10.5811/cpcem.2017.6.34778

[16] Ross/Moore. Diagnostic Imaging: Spine. Third ed. Philadelphia, USA: Elsevier; 2015

[17] Shi J, Jia L, Yuan W, Shi GD, Ma B, Wang B, et al. Clinical classification of

cauda equina syndrome for proper treatment. A retrospective analysis of 39 patients. Acta Orthopedics. 2010;**81**(3): 391-395. DOI: 10.3109/17453674.2010.483985

[18] Peacock JG, Timpone VM. Doing more with less: Diagnostic accuracy of CT in suspected Cauda Equina syndrome. American Journal of Neuroradiology. 2017;**38**(2):391-397. DOI: 10.3174/ajnr.A4974

[19] Yousif S, Musa A, Ahmed A, Abdelhai A. Correlation between findings in physical examination, magnetic resonance imaging, and nerve conduction studies in lumbosacral radiculopathy caused by lumbar intervertebral disc herniation. 2020;**2020**:9719813. DOI: 10.1155/2020/9719813

[20] Qureshi A, Sell P. Cauda equina syndrome treated by surgical decompression. The influence of time on surgical outcome. European Spine Journal. 2007;**16**:2143-2151

[21] Domen PM, Hofman PA, van Santbrink H, et al. Predictive value of clinical characteristics in patients with suspected cauda equina syndrome. European Neurology. 2009;**16**(3):416-419

[22] Pedowitz RA, Garfin SR, Massie JB, et al. Effects of magnitude and duration of compression on spinal nerve root conduction. Spine (Phila PA). 1992;**17**: 194-199

[23] Rooney A, Statham PF, Stone J. Cauda equina syndrome with normal MR imaging. Journal of Neurology. 2009;**256**(5):721-725

[24] Gleave JR, MacFarlane R. Prognosis for recovery of bladder function following lumbar central disc prolapse. British Journal of Neurosurgery. 1990;**4**: 205-209

Chapter 3

Prevalence of Upper Limb Pain in Spinal Cord Injury: A Systematic Review

Adrienne McCann, Daniel Kerr and Mary P.A. Hannon-Fletcher

Abstract

A systematic review was undertaken to evaluate and critically appraise literature pertaining to prevalence and treatment of upper limb pain in the spinal cord injured (SCI) population using manual wheelchair. Data extraction tables were compiled, then an in-depth data on the types of injury, level of injury, type of wheelchair used, type of treatment sought and the impact on Activities of Daily Living were recorded. A Quality Assessment Tool for Observational Cohort and Cross-Sectional Studies tool was used to critically appraise the quality of studies included in this review. 994 papers in total were screened, 46 full text studies were assessed with 14 studies included in the final synthesis: four cohort studies and ten cross-sectional studies. Shoulder pain was the most common type of pain reported (30–71%) followed by wrist, hand, and elbow. Functional limitations reported because of upper limb pain included interference with mobilizing, transferring, and Activities of Daily Living, primarily personal care tasks. There is clear evidence that upper limb pain is prevalent in the SCI manual wheelchair using population which impacts on functional tasks. Further research is required to explore the perceptions of those with upper limb pain and techniques used to manage pain.

Keywords: spinal cord injury, upper limb pain, manual wheelchair users, Musculoskeletal (MSK) pain, upper limb pain management

1. Introduction

Participant with Spinal cord injury (SCI) have been reported to experience premature or accelerated aging in several organ systems in the SCI population compared to the aged matched general population [1]. In addition, they report that chronic pain and other health conditions increases with the duration of SCI. The primary complications that can occur in the short and long term after SCI include musculoskeletal (MSK) pain, muscle atrophy, pressure sores, infections, and respiratory issues [2].

The scope of this review is in relation to Musculoskeletal (MSK) pain, specifically of the upper limb (**Figure 1**). For the purpose of this study, upper limb pain refers to pain or inflammation of the neck, shoulder, elbow, wrist, or fingers as well as the corresponding muscles, ligaments and tendons. There is a substantial amount of

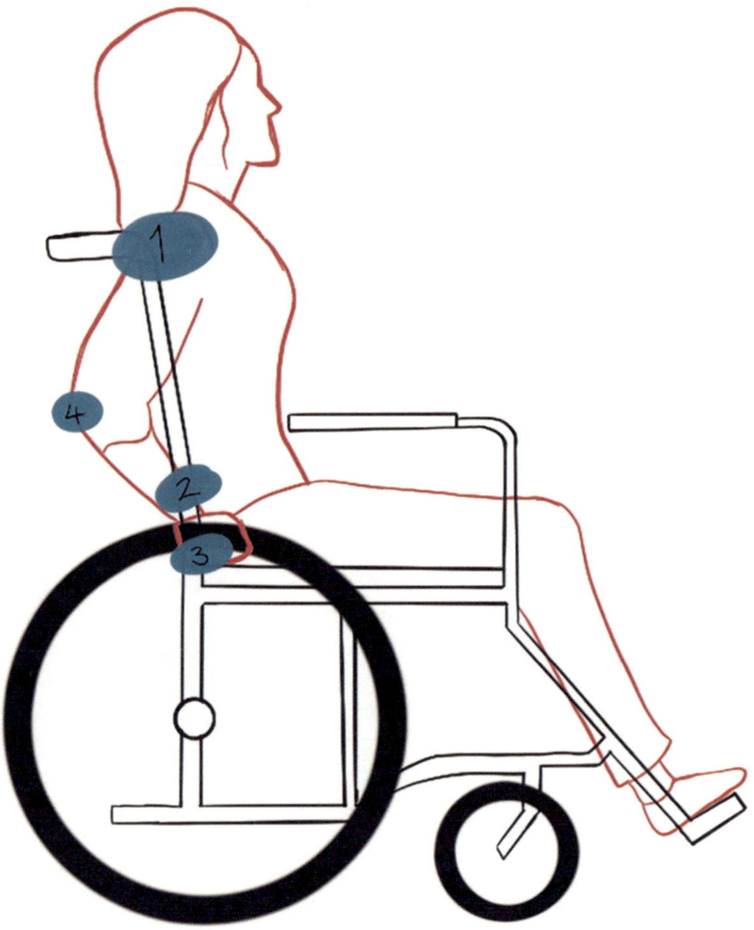

Figure 1.
Prevalence of upper limb pain in the spinal cord injured (SCI) population using manual wheelchair. Adapted from: incountryvalueoman.net. Reproduced with the kind permission of Leda Bug (@art_and_spacecrafts). 1: Shoulder; 2: Wrist; 3: Hand; 4: Elbow.

literature in the area documenting the prevalence of these conditions. Injuries such as shoulder, neck and back pain resulting from poor wheeling practice in the long-term are documented in both those who began wheeling as adults and as children [3–5]. Between 49% and 73% of SCI manual wheelchair users develop carpal tunnel syndrome and between 31% and 71% report shoulder pain [6]. This may have serious implications for functional mobility, sleep and living life independently [7].

Management of upper limb pain may prove difficult due to the nature of the treatment. In many cases relative rest may be required for the upper limb to recover however this may prove problematic as the upper extremity is used for mobility on a daily basis [8]. Pain can contribute to overall poorer health in the SCI population and has been shown to have a negative effect on both physical and psychological aspects of a person's wellbeing [9]. Further long-term pain that is chronic in nature has also been associated with low mood and depressive symptoms in the SCI population [10].

2. Aim

The overall aim of this review is to examine the literature in relation to prevalence of upper limb pain, pain sites reported, treatments availed of and causation of injuries. This review follows the Preferred Reporting Items for Systematic Reviews and Meta-Analyses (PRISMA) guidelines [11].

3. Methods

3.1 Search and study selection

A search was conducted between January–February 2019 for studies reporting on the prevalence of upper limb injuries or pain, in manual wheelchair users with an SCI. Medline (1966 – February 2019), CINAHL (1982 – February 2019), OVID (1966 – February 2019) and PubMed (1971 to February 2019) databases were searched using the terms "spinal cord injur* or SCI" combined with "wrist", "elbow", "shoulder", "neck", "upper limb", "carpal tunnel", "rotator cuff", "parapleg*", and "mobil*", "ambulation", "propel", and "pain". Further literature was obtained by exploring reference lists of papers identified in this search. Each title was screened by a single reviewer for relevance and added to the shortlist if it met the inclusion criteria or if further clarification was required, the abstract or entire paper was reviewed.

3.2 Inclusion and exclusion criteria

Studies were included if they were peer reviewed research studies written in the English language, that directly reported on prevalence of upper limb pain in SCI. Studies were required to include participants with a traumatic SCI only and use a manual wheelchair full time. Other causations of SCI were excluded such as infection or insufficient blood flow, as in these cases participants may regain function and therefore fluctuating prevalence rates of upper limb pain may be observed. Any prevalence rates reported in these studies may be skewed by a participant regaining function or not requiring a wheelchair for mobility purpose therefore would not be an accurate reflection of the true prevalence rates. Studies primarily including wheelchair athletes were also excluded as it is common for athletes to have higher level of activities compared to a sedentary population and may therefore report higher levels of prevalence rates that could not be generalized to the wider SCI population.

3.3 Data collection process

Data extraction tables were compiled (Appendix 1) and included study design, objective, sample size, classification of SCI, type of injury/pain reported, outcome measures used and results of each article. Further in-depth data on the types of injury recorded, level of SCI, type of wheelchair used, type of treatment sought (if applicable) and the impact on ADLs, were also recorded.

3.4 Study quality appraisal

The National Heart, Lung, and Blood Institute (NHLBI) Quality Assessment Tool for Observational Cohort and Cross-Sectional Studies tool was used to critically appraise the quality of studies included in this review. The tool is a widely accepted tool used for appraising observational studies and is particularly useful in identifying methods applied to minimize bias in research literature [12]. The tool itself is a 14-item scale, with each question scored as "yes" or "no". If an item on the checklist cannot be clearly identified, the scorer can assign "cannot determine", "not applicable" or "not relevant". The tool has been designed as a checklist rather than a scoring scale specifically, however, can be used as guidance in determining the methodological quality of studies. All studies were retrieved and reviewed by a single researcher (AMC).

4. Results

The systematic search returned 994 papers in total (**Figure 2**: PRISMA Flow Diagram). Two additional papers were found via hand search and review of relevant reference lists in the subject area. Forty-six studies were selected for further reading. After reviewing the full text studies, 31 studies were excluded after not meeting one or more of the inclusion criteria. The most common inclusion criteria not met was the involvement of part time manual wheelchair users, elite wheelchair athletes or studies not specific to upper limb or extremity injury in the SCI population. The total number of studies included in this review was 15 papers.

Key results for all studies are summarized in Appendix 1. Four studies comprised of cohort methodologies [3, 13–15] following patients for 3 years, 5 years, 18 months and 1-year post SCI rehabilitation respectively. The remaining 11 studies were cross-sectional in design [16–26]. Five studies investigated the prevalence of upper limb pain alone and the remaining 10 studies, included the impact on functional activities.

4.1 Demographic results

Demographic details from each study are outlined in the appendix (Appendix 1). Studies are discussed in further detail below.

4.2 Recruitment

Studies were primarily conducted in the United States of America (USA), (n = 9), two studies conducted in the Netherlands, two in Australia, one in Sweden and one in Israel. Recruitment of participants was primarily conducted via hospital discharge lists (n = 7). Ballinger et al. [13], additionally advertised their study with local radio stations and Boninger et al. [17], advertised with known wheelchair vendors to improve recruitment. 19 Eriks-Hoogland et al. [19], Silfverskiold & Waters [15] and Van Drongelen et al. [3], recruited participants while they were undergoing initial inpatient rehabilitation. Pentland & Twomey [22, 23] stated participants were recruited from the community however it is not clear whether this may have been via discharge lists, advertisements in the media or any other approach. Escobedo et al. [20] and Sie et al. [25] recruited participants directly on attending a routine medical examination at an outpatient appointment as part of their SCI rehabilitation. The remaining studies [16, 18] do not state explicitly where participants were recruited from.

Research study settings refers to where the study took place. Settings were classified as either inpatient, outpatient or community based. Five studies were community based [21–24, 26]. Four studies were outpatient based [18–20, 25]. Two studies were

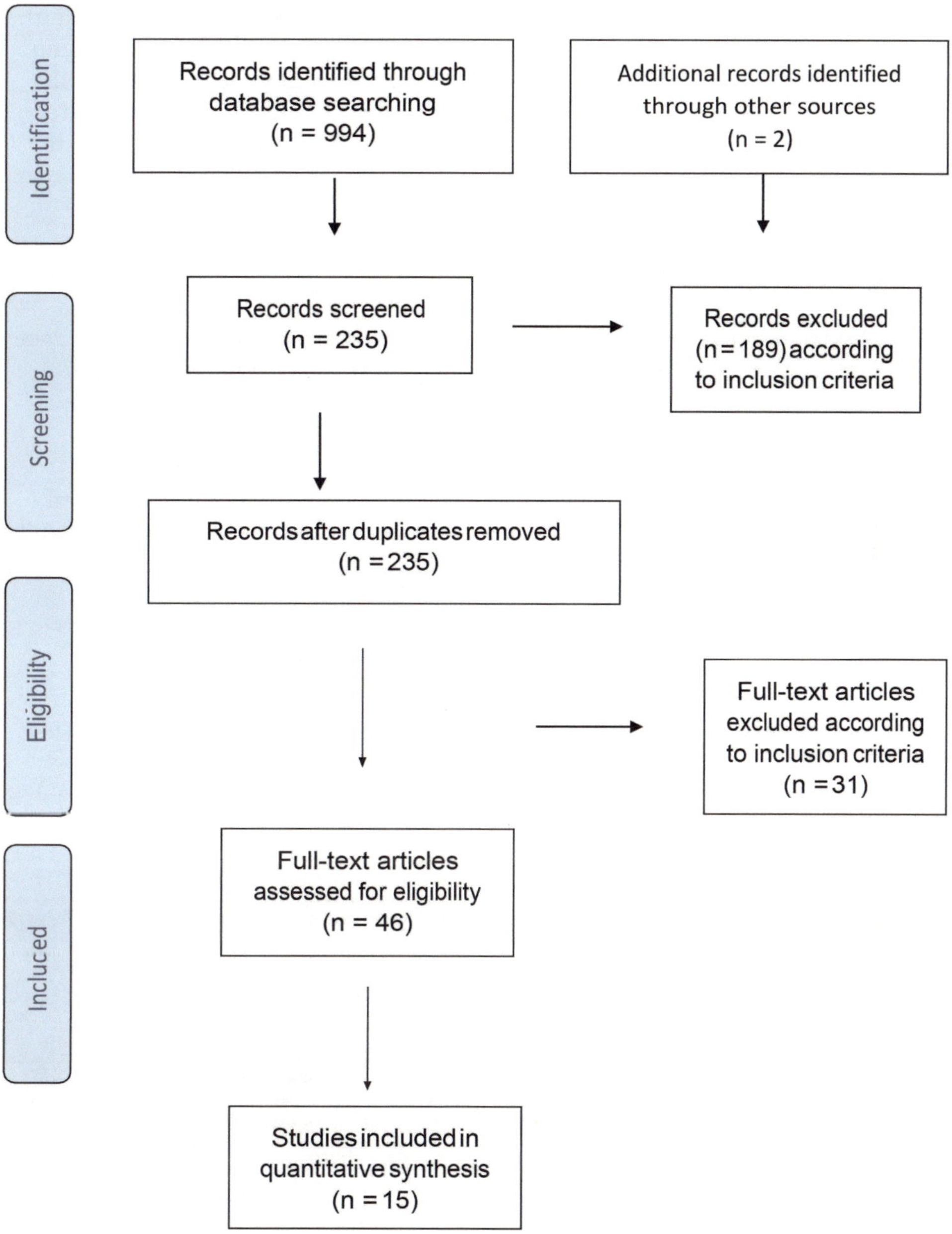

Figure 2.
PRISMA flow diagram.

inpatient based [3, 15], and three availed of a combination of community and outpatient settings [13, 17, 19]. Recruitment methods and setting were unclear for one study [16].

4.3 Response rates

Response rates were detailed in five studies: 76.5% [18], 86%, [19], 46% [21], 63% [24] and 66% [26]. Ballinger et al. [13], reported an oversubscription to their study;

661 participants responded with the authors choosing a sample of 140 participants. Escobedo et al. [20] and Sie et al. [25] used a sample of convenience from patients attending routine outpatient appointments and therefore all patients who met the inclusion criteria were included. The remaining studies did not list response rates specifically, however Eriks-Hoogland et al. [19] reported 60 patients were lost to follow up: 43% dropout rate at the end of the five- year study. The remaining cohort studies do not list details relating to dropout rates or participant retention.

4.4 Sample sizes

Sample sizes ranged from 11 participants [22] to 669 participants [21] in a cross sectional study. Sample sizes for each individual study are outlined in Appendix.

4.5 Age

The youngest participant in all studies was aged 17 years [15], with the oldest participant aged 78 years [20]. Eight studies included age range and mean, six studies reported mean age and one study to record age range [19]. The breakdown of reporting methods for age are outlined below in **Table 1**.

4.6 Gender

Two of the older studies did not provide data relating to gender of participants included in their studies [25, 26]. Three studies used a sample composed of male participants only [16, 20, 22]. The remaining studies all reported a higher percentage of male participants compared to female participants as is reflected in the wider

Reporting method	Author	Age
Studies reporting age range and mean	Aljure et al. [16]	Range = 20–73 years, mean = 47.8
	Ballinger et al. [13]	Range = 19–73 years, mean = 37
	Eriks-Hoogland et al. [14]	Range = 18–66 years, mean = 34
	Escobedo et al. [20]	Range = 40–78 years, mean = 59
	Gironda et al. [21]	Range = 20–65 years, mean = 50.6
	Sie et al. [25]	Range = 17–71 years, mean = 37.4
	Silfverskiold & Waters [15]	Range = 17–40 years, mean = 25
	Subbarao et al. [26]	Range = 21–77 years, mean = 53
Studies reporting mean age only	Boninger et al. [17]	35 years
	Dalyan et al. [18]	42.2 years ± 12
	Pentland & Twomey [22]	44.3 years
	Pentland & Twomey [23]	42.9 years
	Samuelsson et al. [24]	49 years ± 18
	van Drongelen et al. [3]	59.6 years
Study reporting age range only	El-Essi et al. [19]	Range = 18–59 years

Table 1.
Reporting of age across studies.

population of SCI patients, where males are twice as likely to suffer an SCI compared to females [27]. This is primarily attributed to the fact men are more likely to take part in high-risk activities such as high-speed driving or dangerous sports [28]. The higher percentage of males in this review may also be attributed to the study design of several studies included. Three studies were conducted as part of the Veterans Affair medical centers in the USA. A higher percentage of males enroll in the military in the USA and therefore the potential cohort of participants recruited from may have been male dominated [29]. Pentland & Twomey [22], were the only study to include a female only sample. Apart from this study, the highest percentage of female participants was 32% [17], albeit a small sample size (n = 32).

4.7 Level of injury

The reporting of level of injury varied widely between studies. The terms quadriplegia and tetraplegia both refer to the same classification of injury and are based on the terminology used by individual authors and reflects differences in language used around the world. For the purpose of this study, the term tetraplegia will be used. Six studies referred to participants as either patients with paraplegia or tetraplegia. Four of these studies included participants with paraplegia only [16, 17, 19, 24]. Sie et al. [25] and Silfverskiold & Waters [15] included participants with tetraplegia and paraplegia; 57% tetraplegia, 43% paraplegia and 66.6% tetraplegia and 33.3% paraplegia respectively.

Ballinger et al. [13] and Eriks-Hoogland et al. [14] both reported level of injury using a combination of the terms high/low paraplegia/tetraplegia and the American Spinal Injury Association (ASIA) Impairment Scale (AIS) levels A-D. Ballinger et al. [13] range included; 5% high tetraplegia, 39% low tetraplegia, 45% paraplegia, 11% ASIA class D. 14 Eriks-Hoogland et al. [14] included 34.1% tetraplegia and AIS class A or B. Escobedo et al. [20] and van Drongelen et al. [3] both list level of injury as ranges; T3-L2 and C2-S5 respectively. The remaining five studies also list level of injury as ranges however provide further details on the percentage of participants within each range.

Dalyan et al. [18] provided the most in-depth detail regarding level of injury; C2-C4 = 14.5%, C5-C8 = 35.5%, T1–5 = 7.9%, T6-T10 = 19.7%, T11-L2 = 21.1% and L3-L4 = 1.3%. Gironda et al. [21] grouped participant level of injury into three ranges: T2-T6 = 34%, T7- T12 = 56.1% and L1-L2 = 9.9%. Similarly, Pentland & Twomey [22, 23] used three ranges, however ranges differ by one level of injury within their groups. In 1991 [23], they reported level of injury as; T1-T5 = 9%, T6-T10 = 18% and T11-L3 = 73%. In 1994 [22], injury level was reported as; T2-T5 = 20%, T6-T10 = 40% and T11-L2 = 40%. Finally, Subbarao et al. [26] grouped the reporting of level of injury into four ranges: C1-C4 = 9.2%, C5 – T1 = 34.6%, T12-L1 = 37.9% and L2 and below = 13.1%. The full range of reporting measures for level of injury can be found below in **Table 2**.

4.8 Time since injury

Time since injury was reported either as the mean years since injury or the range of years since injury. One study only [13] reported time since injury as the age that SCI occurred; mean = 27 years, range = 14–68 years. Four studies reported time since injury as the mean number of years since injury only: mean = 11.5 years [17], 11.8 years ± 8.5 years [18], 26 years [20], 20.3 years ± 11.1 [21]. Three studies included time

Author (year)	Level of SCI
Aljure et al. [16]	*All participants with paraplegia*
Boninger et al. [17]	
El-Essi et al. [19]	
Samuelsson et al. [24]	
Sie et al. [25]	57% tetraplegia, 43% paraplegia
Silfverskiold and Waters [15]	66.6% tetraplegia and 33.3% paraplegia
Ballinger et al. [15]	5% high tetraplegia, 39% low tetraplegia, 45% paraplegia, 11% ASIA class D
Eriks-Hogland et al. [14]	34.1% tetraplegia and AIS class A or B
Escobedo et al. [20]	T3-L2
van Drongelen et al. [3]	C2-S5
Dalyan et al. [18]	C2-C4 = 14.5%, C5-C8 = 35.5%, T1–5 = 7.9%, T6-T10 = 19.7%, T11-L2 = 21.1% and L3-L4 = 1.3%
Gironda et al. [21]	T2-T6 = 34%, T7-T12 = 56.1% and L1-L2 = 9.9%
Pentland & Twomey [23]	T1-T5 = 9%, T6-T10 = 18% and T11-L3 = 73%
Pentland & Twomey [22]	T2-T5 = 20%, T6-T10 = 40% and T11-L2 = 40%
Subbarao et al. [26]	C1-C4 = 9.2%, C5 – T1 = 34.6%, T12-L1 = 37.9% and L2 and below = 13.1%

Table 2.
Reporting measures for level of injury.

since injury as range, 3 months – 42 years [16] and 6–18 months' post SCI [3, 15]. Four studies included both range and mean time since injury; 1–45 years, mean = 17.4 [22], 5–21 years, mean = 15.2 [23], 1–42 years, mean = 12.1 [25] and 21–77 years, mean = 22.8 [26]. Two studies did not report any details regarding time since injury [14, 19].

4.9 Area of upper limb pain

The most common site of pain investigated was the shoulder alone (n = 7). Of these, Boninger et al. [17] aimed to gain insight into the prevalence of shoulder injuries, however the study was primarily focused on identifying rotator cuff tears in patients with paraplegia. Six studies investigated the prevalence of pain on all the upper extremities; [3, 18, 21–23, 25] while 26 Subbarao et al. [26] investigated pain at both the shoulder and wrists. Both Aljure et al. [16] and 20 Escobedo et al. [20] were distinctive in that they investigated the occurrence of an injury rather than a pain site alone. Aljure et al. [16] investigated the prevalence of carpal tunnel syndrome (CTS), while Escobedo et al. [20] investigated the prevalence of RCTs in patients with paraplegia.

4.10 Outcome measures

The primary outcome measure used in all studies was a self-reported questionnaire establishing prevalence and location of pain (n = 11). Interviews were utilized in six studies, either by telephone or face to face, to gather demographic data and data relating to prevalence of upper limb pain and injury. Eleven studies also conducted physical exams to establish prevalence and location of pain. Postal questionnaires were utilized in five studies [18, 19, 21, 24, 26]. Of these, Samuelsson et al. [24] and Subbarao et al. [26] used postal questionnaires as an identification method to invite participants to attend a physical exam to further investigate upper limb pain. Nine studies formulated their own questionnaire; four studies used these to collect data relating to prevalence and location of pain [14, 17, 18, 21] and five studies used these to collect demographic data [3, 22, 23, 25, 26]. No standardized outcome measures were used solely to report prevalence of pain.

4.11 Functional outcome measures

The relationship between upper limb pain and functional limitations was formally assessed in eleven studies [3, 13–21, 26]. Of these, six studies used standardized outcome measures to report functional limitations [3, 13, 14, 19, 21, 24]. An additional two studies formulated their own functional questionnaire based on standardized outcome measures and pilot tested these with steering groups to ensure content and consensual validity was reached [23, 26]. The most commonly used measures were the Functional Impact Measure (FIM) (n = 3), and the Wheelchair User Shoulder Pain Index (WUSPI) (n = 3); both are reliable and valid tools [30, 31]. The FIM is an 18-item questionnaire designed to assess level of disability and patient's change in health status in response to further disability such as pain or medical intervention. The FIM is a well- documented assessment of functional ability and has been used across a wide range of disability cohorts. In comparison, the WUSPI has been designed specifically for the wheelchair using population, however, is only specific to shoulder pain, not the upper extremity in its entirety.

A wide variety of additional standardized outcome measures were used across all studies including; the Craig Handicap Assessment and Reporting Technique (CHART) (n = 1), the Shoulder Rating Questionnaire (SRQ) (n = 1), the Sickness Impact Profile 68 (SIP68) (n = 1), the Physical Activity Scale for Individuals with Physical Disabilities (PASIPD) (n = 1), the Klein and Bell Activities of Daily Living Scale (n = 1), the Canadian Occupational Performance Measure (COPM) (n = 1), and the Constant Murley Scale (n = 1). Of these, the SRQ and Constant Murley Scale are both specific to shoulder pain, while the remainder are generic tools assessing functional tasks. None of the standardized outcome measures are specifically designed for use with patients with an SCI.

4.12 Physical assessments

Physical assessments of dysfunction were utilized in twelve studies. Of these, eleven studies utilized a standardized method of assessment [3, 13–17, 20, 22, 23, 25].

Radiographic imaging was utilized in three studies [13, 17, 20]. Radiographic images were taken following clinical protocols for identification of RCTs [13, 17]. Shoulders were x-rayed in anteroposterior position only [13], while Boninger et al. [17] used additional positions of scapular anteroposterior position and supraspinatus position.

Ballinger et al. [13] also conducted a physical assessment of participants using manual muscle testing and range of movement (ROM). ROM was assessed in three additional studies [14, 22, 23]. Eriks-Hoogland et al. [14] assessed physical ROM via manual muscle testing and completion of the Wheelchair Skills Test. Biomechanical measures were taken using peak power output (POpeak) requiring participants to complete a maximal wheelchair exercise test on a motor-driven treadmill.

Transfers were also assessed using the FIM. Pentland & Twomey [22], assessed ROM at both the shoulder and elbow. Bilateral upper limb function was assessed using concentric isokinetic torque using KinCom II isokinetic dynamometer and Smedley's handheld dynamometer, both which are valid and accurate tools for measuring muscle strength [32, 33]. In comparison, van Drongelen et al. [3] measured muscle strength subjectively as scored by the research assistant. Aljure et al. [16] focusedecifically on the incidence of CTS and assessed this by utilizing electrophysiological studies of the median and ulnar nerves following a standardized protocol [34].

4.13 Prevalence

All studies reported various areas and levels of upper limb pain or injury. Detailed prevalence rates by setting have been outlined in **Table 3**. The most common area of pain reported in the upper limb was the shoulder and the highest prevalence of shoulder pain was 71% [18], unspecified upper limb pain reported was 81% [21], however it is not aligned to any particular structure of the upper limb.

Setting*	Measure	Shoulder	Elbow	Wrist	Hand
Inpatient setting N = 2	*Median*	33%	N/A	N/A	N/A
	Mean	33%	N/A	N/A	N/A
	Highest	56.5%	N/A	N/A	N/A
	Lowest	39%	N/A	N/A	N/A
Outpatient setting N = 4	*Median*	66%	25.5%	33.5%	28%
	Mean	61%	25.2%	33.5%	28%
	Highest	71%	35%	53%	43%
	Lowest	41%	15.5%	14%	13%
Community setting N = 4	*Median*	39%	20%	40%	45%
	Mean	54.3%	20%	33.8%	45%
	Highest	73%	31%	55%	45%
	Lowest	35.6%	9%	6.6%	45%
Community and outpatient N = 2	*Median*	31%	N/A	N/A	N/A
	Mean	31%	N/A	N/A	N/A
	Highest	32%	N/A	N/A	N/A
	Lowest	30%	N/A	N/A	N/A
Range and mean of combined prevalence estimates:		Shoulder	Elbow	Wrist	Hand
		Range = 35.6% - 73% Mean = 44.8%	Range = 9% - 35% Mean = 22.6%	Range = 6.6% - 55% Mean = 33.6%	Range = 13% - 45% Mean = 36.5%

**[16] did not detail the setting of their study and no specific percentages of pain per area were reported in [3], both have therefore been excluded from this table.*

Table 3.
Prevalence of upper limb pain by setting.

Prospective cohort studies were undertaken in 5 studies [3, 13, 14, 18] and they recorded the level of upper limb pain. Ballinger et al. [13], reported an increase of shoulder pain over the 3-year study, and this was more prevalent in men who were older, reported poorer health and had acromioclavicular (AC) joint narrowing as determined by X-ray on first admission to rehabilitation. In contrast to this, van Drongelen et al. [3] reported a decrease in shoulder pain (30%) at the second test point. Muscle strength was significantly inversely related to shoulder pain at the beginning of rehabilitation and body mass index (BMI) was a strong predictor for pain, one year after in-patient rehabilitation. Both [13, 14] reported 32% of participants had limited shoulder ROM and 39% reported pain at the shoulder on discharge from rehabilitation.

Aljure et al. [16] and Escobedo et al. [20] both investigated the prevalence of a specific injury, CTS and RCT respectively. Aljure et al. [16] reported 63% of participants had electrical nerve abnormalities confirming the presence of CTS, while 44.7% also had ulnar nerve neuropathy. Escobedo et al. [20] reported 70% of participants were symptomatic of RCT, with MRI imaging showing 62% full RCTs and 12% partial RCTs. Samuellson et al. [24] was the only study to associate pain with a diagnosis of a condition. Thirty seven percent of participants reported shoulder pain, with findings of muscular atrophy, pain, impingement, and tendinopathy described. The estimated mean prevalence of upper limb pain by outcome measure has been detailed below in **Table 4**.

4.14 Relationship of pain with participant characteristics

The relationship between pain and wheelchair user's characteristics was investigated in thirteen studies. Significant results were reported in nine of these studies. Time since injury was a significant factor in predisposing participants to the development of upper limb pain. More specifically, [15, 21, 22] reported the development of unspecified upper limb pain was significantly associated with length of time since injury and Aljure et al. [16] reported significant incidence of CTS increased with length of time since injury. Level of SCI was significantly related to upper limb pain in two studies [2, 22]. Pentland & Twomey [22] reported pain is significantly associated with participants with paraplegia compared to the able-bodied population, while van Drongelen et al. [3] reported participants with tetraplegia are significantly predisposed to developing upper limb pain compared to participants with paraplegia.

Two studies reported significant relationships between upper limb pain and age [18, 20] although this contradicts findings from three studies who reported no significant correlation between pain and age [22, 24, 26]. Additionally, radiographic results from Boninger et al. [17] found a significant relationship between imaging abnormalities and Body Mass Index (BMI), but not pain.

	Questionnaire element N = 6	Physical Exam N = 3	Radiographic element N = 3	Electrophysiological element N = 1
Mean	52.6%	50.3%	50%	63%
Highest	71%%	73%	70%	63%
Lowest	35.6%	39%	30%	63%

Table 4.
Estimated mean prevalence of upper limb pain by outcome measure.

4.15 Relationship of pain with functional activities

Of the studies reviewed, eight assessed the impact of upper limb pain on functional activities. Dalyan et al. [18], reported the highest level of pain was associated with pressure relieving, transfers, and wheelchair mobility. Gironda et al. [21] similarly to Dalyan et al. [18], reported wheelchair mobility and transportation as the activities resulting in the greatest amount of pain in the upper limb. Further to this, El Essi et al. [19] examined wheelchair mobility to include pushing a wheelchair, propulsion up ramps and outdoor inclines as the primary contributors to upper limb pain. Seventy-four percent reported no limitation during recreational or athletic activities, while the remainder agreed that pain had limited function to varying degrees. Few participants reported seeking treatment for this issue, only 23–35% made changes to their routines and 6–16% had sought assistance from a carer or friend with ADLs due to upper limb pain.

Samuellson et al. [24], used the Canadian Occupational Performance Measure (COPM) to assess the impact on ADLs. From this, issues in 52 areas of occupational performance were associated with upper limb pain, with 54% of these related to self-care. Furthermore, van Drongelen et al. [3] found upper limb pain to be significantly inversely related to functional outcome. Eriks-Hoogland et al. [14] reported limitations of shoulder ROM were significantly associated with the ability to transfer, FIM motor scores and participants returning to work. Pentland & Twomey [22] devised their own questionnaire based on the Barthel Index. Although functional limitations were not formally assessed, participants with pain reported tasks most impeded by pain included work/school, sleep, wheelchair transfers, outdoor wheeling, and driving.

One study included a female only sample [23], participants reported outdoor wheeling as the most difficult task to complete while experiencing pain. Additionally, Ballinger et al. [13] reported men with shoulder pain scored lower CHART and FIM scores, however, this was not statistically significant.

4.16 Study quality appraisal

Appendix 2 provides details on the quality of the studies. There were four cohort studies and eleven cross-sectional studies. The cohort studies scored moderately well on the checklist with all scoring positively on over half of the criteria [3, 14, 15, 18]. The remaining cross-sectional studies scored lower overall due to several biases relating to study design and analysis of data. In relation to the studies composed of a radiographic element, only one study blinded the reporting radiographer to participants [17]. Escobedo et al. [20] stated three observers interpreted the MRI results however it is unclear if they were blinded or what level of expertise they held. Four studies did not include any standardized outcome measures therefore questioning the validity and reliability of their results [18, 22, 23, 25]. Self-reporting questionnaires are also a limitation as they are likely to present an over endorsement bias, where participants answer questions relating to their health in an enthusiastic manner, often over reporting the extent of their pain or injury [35].

Physical assessments were conducted in twelve studies with five of these studies following standard protocols for the reporting of muscle strength and ROM [3, 15, 16, 24, 26]. Although, van Drongelen et al. [3] used a standardized protocol to conduct manual muscle testing, muscle force was subjectively measured by the research assistant therefore impacting the quality and objectivity of results reported. Pentland & Twomey [22, 23], were the only two studies to use mechanical devices to measure muscle strength via use of a dynamometer. Dynamometers are well documented as accurate devices in reporting grip strength and therefore add to the methodological quality of these studies [36].

Sample size varied greatly across all studies. A larger sample size increases the validity of results as it reduces the chance of error that results occurred because of another reason and not the hypothesis in question. Four sample sizes included over one hundred participants however it was unclear if power calculations were conducted to ensure generalizability of results. The smallest sample sizes were observed in [23] 11 participants and [17] 28 participants. A smaller sample size increases the risk of error in applying results to the wider SCI population and therefore these results should be interpreted with caution.

Recruitment bias refers to the methods utilized by studies for inclusion of participants. Several studies recruited participants from specific hospitals catering for different diseases or conditions. Five studies recruited participants from Veteran Affairs Hospitals [13, 17, 20, 21, 26] who provide care specifically to Veterans and their families. Recruitment bias may exist where participants may not be an accurate representation of the wider SCI population, or it may result in an uneven representation of the wider population as the hospital caters to a specific population of SCI patients.

4.17 Causation of secondary musculoskeletal (MSK) injuries

The etiology of upper limb pain was primarily attributed to the overuse of the upper limb during wheelchair propulsion and transfers in twelve studies. Functional activities which exacerbated pain the most included outdoor wheeling, ramps/inclines, wheelchair transfers and domestic ADLs (DADLs). Gironda et al. [21] concluded that although the overuse of the upper limb contributed to injury or pain, it was not sufficient in explaining the development of pain itself. They stated the development, persistence and exacerbation of pain is further aggravated by functional activities; however, injuries would be best understood in the context of a theoretical model to understand the person as a whole.

Similarly, Subbarao et al. [26] reported that not all pain can be attributed to the overuse of the upper limb alone. They reported that acute trauma to a joint or structure in the upper limb could cause early pain, while cumulative trauma may result in late onset of injuries. Incorrect loading of joints or abnormal movement patterns were viewed as the primary causation factors of upper limb pain in two studies [15, 24].

Samuelsson et al. [24] discussed the anatomical positioning of wheelchair users during wheelchair propulsion. He concluded the kyphotic position wheelchair users adopt while propelling places further strain on the shoulder joint, depressing the acromial process, and changing the facing of the glenoid fossa, thus resulting in pain and injury. Similarly, Silfverskiold & Waters [15] attributed the causation of injury to abnormal glenohumeral motion during active or passive ROM of the shoulder joint. Boninger et al. [17] was the only study to attribute the causation of pain to increased BMI in SCI participants. They reported an increased BMI resulted in increased weight for participants during wheelchair propulsion and transfers, thus placing further strain on the upper limb joints and structures.

Distinctly, only two studies attempted to distinguish the type of pain experienced by participants. Neuropathic pain is a common occurrence in the SCI population where pain occurs below or surrounding the level of injury. Both Eriks-Hoogland et al. [14] and van Drongelen et al. [3] attempted to distinguish between neuropathic pain and upper limb pain. Both used self-reporting questionnaires advising participants to report only pain they experienced because of trauma or injury, not directly related to their injury. It is not always possible to distinguish between both types of pain and the use of self-reported questionnaires placed the onus on participants to decipher this individually. It is therefore difficult to confirm if pain that was neuropathic in origin was included in their analysis.

4.18 Treatments sought

Only four studies reported on treatments availed of by participants experiencing upper limb pain [18, 21, 22, 25]. Dalyan et al. [18] provided the most in-depth detail relating to treatments, stating 63% sought medical intervention on experiencing pain. Of this, 90% received either physiotherapy, pharmacological treatment or massage, and home modifications or joint protection education was sought by 27% of participants. Joint protection education was reported to be most beneficial by 63.3% of participants, however it is unclear when, or who delivered this. Twenty-six percent of participants also found home modifications useful.

Both Gironda et al. [21] and Sie et al. [25] detailed how 43% and 30% of participants respectively used opiate medications daily, which provided only moderate relief. Pentland & Twomey [22] discussed treatment options availed of by participants and found that many participants were fearful of seeking treatments such as steroid injections, surgery, or hospital admission due to the invasive nature of such. The final treatment option which was discussed was that of resting the upper limb, however participants felt this was unachievable.

5. Discussion

The results from this systematic literature review highlight varying prevalence rates of upper limb pain across 15 studies. The shoulder was the primary pain site investigated by studies, with three studies investigating prevalence of pain of the upper limb in its entirety.

Prevalence rates ranged from 11–81% and differed by reporting measures, outcome measures utilized, recruitment methods, level of injury of participants, time since injury and age. Little is currently known regarding prevalence rates of upper limb pain in SCI, however it is anticipated this review will highlight the variety of research undertaken and gaps in knowledge relating to upper limb pain in the SCI population.

There was considerable variation in the method of data collection across all studies. The heterogeneity of studies implies difficulty in drawing overall conclusions from the studies included [37]. The reported pain values vary from 11% -81%; no clustering of prevalence rates was noted suggesting the samples are heterogeneous. The varying levels of SCI were not consistently recorded. Some studies used the ASIA scale, some studies stated either participants with tetraplegia or paraplegia, and some studies stratified participants based on the medical level of injury reported. The lack of standard criteria defining level of injury in each study offers minimal help in explaining between-sample differences thus making it difficult to report results applicable to the wider SCI population.

The use of self-reported questionnaires was the most prevalent methodology utilized on the basis that they are cost effective and easy to administer. Self-reported questionnaires have been used widely across healthcare research to obtain prevalence rates, health status and health services accessed [38]. Self-reported questionnaires are useful when the data required is not normally collected via audits or medical practice or when database analysis is deemed too expensive or time consuming to conduct [39]. Despite the widespread use of these, there is little consensus regarding the accuracy of information reported and the validity of findings [40]. Potential bias lies in the over or under-reporting by participants such as recall timeframe where participants may suffer memory decay. Literature shows an increased number of hospital or healthcare visits results in an under-reporting of the number of visits; the more often they occur, the less memorable they are to participants [41–43]. Over endorsement bias may also exist where participants may under or over-report pain to please their healthcare professional or as an incentive to be included in a research study. Although this questions the validity of results, self-reported questionnaires are often the only option to obtain data when it is not recorded elsewhere.

A systematic review investigated prevalence of pain in cancer patients [44]. They found the use of self-reported measures were more reliable than medically documented symptoms, as pain was only recorded by 10% of oncologists, resulting in the underestimation of the prevalence of pain. This is in part due to the complex nature of cancer where pain may not have been a priority for the physician to assess. It is reasonable to draw comparisons between the recording of pain in cancer populations and SCI populations as both conditions are complex in nature and potentially have more critical issues associated with their condition to report. Individuals who are diagnosed with a condition or illness are also less likely to report abnormal sensations or health related issues as they attribute these to the disease itself [45].

Muhajarine et al. [46] conducted a study on individuals with hypertension and compared the efficacy of self-reporting questionnaires to that of an able-bodied population. They reported that participants with hypertension were less likely to report abnormal issues via use of a self-reported questionnaire in comparison to attending a physical assessment by a healthcare professional. Similarly, to patients with an SCI, it could be argued that they felt this complaint was not significant enough to formally report in a questionnaire, however a face-to-face consultation may identify pain via a physical assessment or may allow healthcare professionals to probe further during consultations.

Within this current review, three studies utilized radiographic imaging to explore the pathology of pain and three studies also invited participants to attend for a physical assessment of their pain. The variance in methodology may have contributed to the variance in prevalence rates reported. A physical exam by a trained healthcare professional may provide objective reporting of injuries however a lack of standardized outcome measures utilized by studies resulted in data lacking validity and reliability.

Physical assessments of pain may also be deemed as invasive for participants who experience pain, and an additional burden lies on the participant in attending appointments and undergoing tests for the purpose of a research study. For the research team, both the use of physical assessments and radiographic imaging are time consuming and require expert knowledge and a number of assessors in order to ensure reliability and validity of results. Taking all of the above literature into account, the use of a self-reported questionnaire in the SCI population is feasible and cost effective, however may not be sufficient in accurately reporting the prevalence of pain or treatments availed of. Therefore, it could be argued that participant reported prevalence rates could be confirmed by accessing patient medical notes to determine specifically what pain they reported, how often it was reported, and treatments prescribed for the management of their pain.

The reporting of pain may also lead to questions around the validity of results in this review. Research evidence shows that of those with SCI who have experienced chronic pain, 40% of patient's pain is neuropathic in origin [47]. Neuropathic pain (NP) can occur above, at, or below the level of SCI and is commonly described as sensations of "burning", "stabbing", or "electric shock like" [2, 48]. Given the expressed unsettling and untreatable nature of the pain by the patients themselves, it is not surprising that NP is one of the most frequently reported and most difficult to treat secondary health conditions associated with SCI [49]. The chronicity and prevalence of pain is strongly associated with an increase in hospital visits and utilization of medical services [50, 51] NP is also quite difficult to distinguish from musculoskeletal pain. NP can occur at or below the level of injury, however in incomplete SCI, MSK pain can also occur at these sites thus making it difficult to determine the origin of pain.

Within this review, only two studies defined the origin of the type of pain experienced. Although some studies linked pain experience to functional activities, it is difficult to decipher whether the pain experienced is related to the level of injury or whether the pain is from functional activity alone [52]. The use of self-reported outcome measures further confounds this, putting the onus on participants themselves to make this distinction, which may prove difficult.

The causation of pain was attributed to the overuse of the upper limb in twelve studies. Wheelchair users rely on the upper limb for mobilizing on a daily basis so it is unsurprising that this plays a role in the development of pain. Two studies referred to the development of pain stemming from anatomical positions adopted during specific wheelchair related activities. With such a small number of studies reporting this, it is difficult to determine if this is the sole source of pain or if there are other variables involved. Further research relating to the biomechanical movement patterns of wheelchair use may help explore the etiology of injuries. Furthermore, wheelchair skills training could play a role in educating patients on joint protection during activities [26].

Pain was most exacerbated by outdoor wheeling, propelling up ramps or inclines and wheelchair transfers. Education around energy efficient propulsion techniques or use of assistive technology to aid transfers may prove beneficial, however there is little literature to confirm this. Only four studies discussed the type of treatments the participants availed of. Only one study [22] further investigated the use of treatments and found participants were fearful of seeking invasive treatments for relief, and rest was deemed unachievable. The question remains, what treatments are available, what are the advantages/disadvantages of each and how effective are they at relieving pain? Further research is also required to understand the implications of pain for participants. How does pain affect their day to day lives with work/school activities, sleep, personal care tasks, domestic ADLs, childcare, or other psychosocial elements of their lives.

To the author's knowledge, only one study from the United Kingdom (UK) has addressed the prevalence of upper limb pain in the SCI population. Nichols et al. [53] was one of the earliest studies to document the phenomenon of overuse injuries in the SCI population, however, was excluded from this review on the basis that powered wheelchair users were included in the sample. Statistics relating to wheelchair use in Northern Ireland are limited, with the most recent figures estimating approximately 30,000 of the 1.8 million population of Northern Ireland classified as wheelchair users [54]. This equates to 1.3% of the Northern Ireland population which is below the UK National average of 2%. It is not clear how accurate the regional figures are, and they may not reflect the true situation. Northern Ireland has a strong history of conflict, most noticeably "The Troubles" which lasted from 1960 to 1998, resulting in over 47,000 individuals injured and 500 severely injured [55].

Indeed, a similar country with a history of conflict (but on a greater scale) took place in the Gaza Strip, Israel [19]. They hypothesized that the number of persons with an SCI in the Gaza Strip increased due to the conflict during the Al Asqa Intifada (2000–2005). Excessive force and the use of explosive devices was prevalent in war torn areas resulting in widespread casualties. Similar to El-Essi et al. [19], it is reasonable to argue that the number of wheelchair users or those with an SCI is potentially under-reported in Northern Ireland. From 1960 to 1998 there were 36,923 shootings, 16,209 bombings and approximately 47,541 people were injured in Northern Ireland (Conflict Archive on the Internet last modified 1/02/18). Those who may have been injured during the troubles 10–50 years ago are now long-term wheelchair users. With length of time since injury significantly associated with the development of upper limb pain, and a potential greater sample of wheelchair users in Northern Ireland as a result of The Troubles, it is reasonable to hypothesize that Northern Ireland will have a higher SCI population and specifically a higher percentage of upper limb pain as documented in long-term wheelchair users. There is currently no literature documenting the prevalence of upper limb pain in the SCI population of Northern Ireland, a significant gap in knowledge considering the history of the country.

5.1 Review limitations

This review was limited in that only studies specifically referring to upper limb pain were included. Studies reporting on generalized pain in the SCI population were excluded as they were not directly relevant to the research question. Other limitations of the study were due to the exclusion of studies not written in the English language. Studies specifically focused on wheelchair athletes were also excluded as this population experience a higher level of physical activity and the potential for sporting injuries may skew results rather than reporting of injuries sustained by manual wheelchair use alone.

6. Conclusion

The increasing number of people with an SCI living longer and healthier lives comes with a consequence of secondary musculoskeletal impairments. The most common site of pain investigated was the shoulder. Varying reporting measures of age, time since injury, level of injury and standardized outcome measures hampered the comparison of the overall prevalence rates of upper limb pain. Little is currently known of the etiology of upper limb pain, treatments available for upper limb pain or how pain affects sufferers on a daily basis. A uniform measurement of upper limb pain specific to the SCI population would be useful in comparing prevalence rates, however none currently exist. A basic pain data set (International Spinal Cord Injury Basic Pain Data Set, ISCIPDS) has been developed within the framework of the International Spinal Cord Injury data sets with the purpose of facilitating consistent collection and reporting of pain in the SCI population [56, 57] however, it is not specific to the reporting of upper limb pain. Future research should focus on what treatments are available and most effective at treating upper limb pain in SCI, specifically in Northern Ireland where an underestimated population of long-term wheelchair users may exist.

Conflict of interest

The authors declare no conflict of interest.

Appendix 1: Study Characteristics.

Reference	Design	N =	Aims	Follow up	Method	Outcome measures	ADLs
[16]	Cross sectional	47 (91 hands)	To assess the prevalence of carpel tunnel syndrome in patients with paraplegia	N/A	Electro physiological studies of the median and ulnar nerves Physical exam	Standardized protocol for conducting tests according to Johnson 1980	No
[15]	Cohort	89	To determine if shoulder pain and ROM problems can be predicted by demographic, injury related, body weight and radiographic data over 3 years	3 years	Radiographic assessment of shoulders in anteroposterior position Questionnaires Physical exam	FIM CHART	Yes
[17]	Cross sectional	28	To use magnetic resonance imaging (MRI), plain radiographs, questionnaire and physical exam to gain insight into the prevalence of shoulder disorders	N/A	MRI X-ray Questionnaire Physical exam	MRI clinical protocol for identification of rotator cuff tears (RCT) X-rayed in AP, scapular AP and supraspinatus position	No
[18]	Cross sectional	130	To determine the frequency and severity of UE pain and its association with functional activities	N/A	Postal questionnaire	Non-validated questionnaire	Yes
[19]	Cross sectional	80	Examine the prevalence of shoulder pain and its effects on ADLs	N/A	Interview Questionnaires	WUSPI Shoulder Rating Questionnaire (SRQ)	Yes
[14]	Cohort	138	Examine whether MSK shoulder pain at first discharge are associated with ADL restriction at 5 years	5 years	Questionnaire Physical exam 3 wheelchair related tests	Physical Activity Scale for Individuals with Physical Disabilities (PASIPD) 2 subscales from the sickness Impact Profile 68 (SIP68) (mobility range and social behavior scales)	Yes

[20]	**Cross sectional**	**37**	**To use MR imaging to evaluate the prevalence and extent of rotator cuff tears in patients with paraplegia**	**N/A**	**MRI (3 observers to interpret results) Scanned patients in supine position with arms adducted and the humerus head in neutral**	**MRI machine (Gyroscan ACS-2)**	**No**
[21]	Cross sectional	669	Examine the prevalence and intensity of pain and associated patient characteristics in paraplegia	N/A	Questionnaire of medical history Questionnaire	WUSPI	Yes
[53]	Cross sectional	517		N/A	Postal survey		No
[22]	Cross sectional	52	Describe the effects of longterm paraplegia and wheelchair use on upper limb function	N/A	Physical exam – physical performance and parameters of upper limb function Interview Questionnaire	Upper extremity isokinetic and grip strength, pain and active ROM using KinCom II isokinetic dynamometer	Yes
[23]	Cross sectional	11	To compare upper limb function and pain in wheelchair using women with paraplegia to a matched able bodied sample	N/A	Physical exam – physical performance and parameters of upper limb function Interview Questionnaire	Upper extremity isokinetic and grip strength, pain and active ROM using KinCom II isokinetic dynamometer Smedley's hand held dynamometer	Yes
[24]	Cross sectional	56	To describe the consequences of shoulder pain on activity and	N/A	Questionnaire WUSPI Interview	WUSPI Constant Murley Scale Klein and Bell ADL index	Yes
			participation in SCI wheelchair users with paraplegia		**Constant Murley Scale Klein and Bell ADL index COPM Physical exam**	**COPM**	
[25]	Cross sectional	239	To determine the prevalence of upper extremity pain in outpatients with SCI	N/A	Questionnaire Interview Physical exam (Pts offered physical exam following pain)	2 point discrimination and Semmes- Weinstein monofilament testing	No
[15]	Cohort	60	To determine the incidence of non-traumatic shoulder pain and associated functional disability during the first 18 months after SCI	18 months	Physical exam following standard protocol at 6 months and then between 6 and 18 months following this	Own questionnaire Physical exam	Yes

			participation in SCI wheelchair users with paraplegia		**Constant Murley Scale Klein and Bell ADL index COPM Physical exam**	**COPM**	
					Functional disability questionnaire		
[26]	Cross sectional	451	To identify the prevalence of chronic wrist and shoulder pain, to determine which activities caused or exacerbated pain and assess functional and emotional responses and how pain might be reduced.	N/A	Review of medical records Postal survey Physical exam (n = 30) Interviewed prior to physical exam Included completing functional tasks transferring, propelling and dressing upper bodies	Own questionnaire previously pilot tested If pain reported in questionnaire participants were interviewed and then physical exam using standardized evaluation sheet	Yes
[3]	Cohort	169	To study MSK UE pain during and after rehabilitation in wheelchair using participants with SCI and its relationship with lesion characteristics, muscle strength and functional outcome	1 year	4 test occasions Physical exam MSK pain questionnaire Manual muscle testing (MMT)	Lesion and personal characteristics assessed by physician Used standardized questionnaire MMT conducted in standardized positions Muscle force measured subjectively by research assist. FIM	Yes

ROM = Range of Movement; FIM = Functional Index Measure; CHART = Craig Handicap Assessment and Reporting Technique; MRI = Magnetic Resonance Imaging; RCT = Rotator Cuff Tear; AP = Anteroposterior; UE = Upper Extremity; ADLs = Activities of Daily Living; SRQ = Shoulder Rating Questionnaire; PASIPD = Physical Activity Scale for Individuals with Physical Disabilities; SIP68 = Sickness Impact Scale; WUSPI = Wheelchair Users Shoulder Pain Index; SCI = Spinal Cord Injury; COPM = Canadian Occupational Performance Measure; MSK = Musculoskeletal; MMT = Manual Muscle Testing.

Author details

Adrienne McCann[1], Daniel Kerr[2] and Mary P.A. Hannon-Fletcher[3]*

1 Maynooth University, Kildare, Ireland

2 School of Health Sciences, Ulster University, Newtownabbey, Ireland

3 School of Biomedical Science, Ulster University, Coleraine, Ireland

*Address all correspondence to: mp.hannon@ulser.ac.uk

References

[1] Pope AM, Tarlov AR. Institute of Medicine. Disability in America: Toward a National Agenda for Prevention. Washington, DC: The National Academies Press; 1991. DOI: 10.17226/1579

[2] Sezer N, Akkus A, Ugurlu FG. Chronic complications of spinal cord injury. World Journal of Orthopedics. 2015;**6**(1):24-33

[3] Van Drongelen S, De Groot S, Veeger H, Angenot E, Dallmeijer A, Post M, et al. Upper extremity musculoskeletal pain during and after rehabilitation in wheelchair-using persons with a spinal cord injury. Spinal Cord. 2006;**44**(3):152-159

[4] Kennedy P, Lude P. Taylor N quality of life, social participation, appraisals and coping post spinal cord injury: A review of four community samples. Spinal Cord. 2006;**44**(2):95-105

[5] Rice I, Impink B, Niyonkuru C, Boninger M. Manual wheelchair stroke characteristics during an extended period of propulsion. Spinal Cord. 2009; **47**(5):413-417

[6] Toosi K, Impink B, Colinger J, Yang J, Koontz A, Boninger M. Correlation between wrist biomechanics and median nerve health parameters in manual wheelchair users. In: American Society of Biomechanics, 34th Annual Meeting. Providence, RI USA: Brown; 18–21 August 2010

[7] Widerström-Noga EG, Felipe-Cuervo E, Yezierski RP. Chronic pain after spinal injury: Interference with sleep and daily activities. Archives of Physical Medicine and Rehabilitation. 2001;**82**(11):1571-1577

[8] Alm M, Saraste H, Norrbrink C. Shoulder pain in persons with thoracic spinal cord injury: Prevalence and characteristics. Journal of Rehabilitation Medicine. 2008;**40**(4):277-283

[9] Ma VY, Chan I, Carruthers KJ. Incidence, prevalence, costs, and impact on disability of common conditions requiring rehabilitation in the United States: Stroke, spinal cord injury, traumatic brain injury, multiple sclerosis, osteoarthritis, rheumatoid arthritis, limb loss, and back pain. Archives of Physical Medicine and Rehabilitation. 2014;**95**(5):986-995

[10] Rintala DH, Loubser PG, Castro J, Hart KA, Fuhrer MJ. Chronic pain in a community-based sample of men with spinal cord injury: Prevalence, severity, and relationship with impairment, disability, handicap, and subjective well-being. Archives of Physical Medicine and Rehabilitation. 1998;**79**(6):604-614

[11] Moher D, Liberati A, Tetzlaff J, Altman GD, PRISMA Group. Preferred reporting items for systematic reviews and meta-analyses: The PRISMA statement. Annals of Internal Medicine. 2009;**151**(4):264-269

[12] Carter BJ. Evidence-based decision-making: Practical issues in the appraisal of evidence to inform policy and practice. Australian Health Review. 2010;**34**(4):435-440

[13] Ballinger DA, Rintala DH, Hart KA. The relation of shoulder pain and range-of-motion problems to functional limitations, disability, and perceived health of men with spinal cord injury: A multifaceted longitudinal study. Archives of Physical Medicine and Rehabilitation. 2000;**81**(12):1575-1581

[14] Eriks-Hoogland I, De Groot S, Snoek G, Stucki G, Post M, Der

Woude V, et al. Association of shoulder problems in persons with spinal cord injury at discharge from inpatient rehabilitation with activities and participation 5 years later. Archives of Physical Medicine and Rehabilitation. 2016;**97**(1):84-91

[15] Silfverskiold J, Waters EL. Shoulder pain and functional disability in spinal cord injury patients. Clinical Orthopaedics and Related Research. 1991;**272**:141-145

[16] Aljure J, Eltorai I, Bradley WE, Lin JE, Johnson B. Carpal tunnel syndrome in paraplegic patients. Spinal Cord. 1985;**23**(3):182-186

[17] Boninger ML, Towers JD, Cooper RA, Dicianno BE, Munin MC. Shoulder imaging abnormalities in individuals with paraplegia. Journal of Rehabilitation Research and Development. 2001;**38**(4):401-408

[18] Dalyan M, Cardenas D, Gerard B. 1999. Upper extremity pain after spinal cord injury. Spinal Cord. 1999;**37**(3): 191-195

[19] El Esse K, El-Shafie JM, Al Hawamdah Z, Zaqout SI. Shoulder pain among rehabilitated spinal cord injured persons using manually propelled wheelchairs in the Gaza strip: A survey. Asia Pacific Disability Rehabilitation Journal. 2012;**23**(2):53-71

[20] Escobedo EM, Hunter JC, Hollister MC, Patten RM, Goldstein B. MR imaging of rotator cuff tears in individuals with paraplegia. AJR. American Journal of Roentgenology. 1997;**168**(4):919-923

[21] Gironda RJ, Clark M, Neugaard B, Nelson A. Upper limb pain in a national sample of veterans with paraplegia. The Journal of Spinal Cord Medicine. 2004; **27**(2):120-127

[22] Pentland W, Twomey l. Upper limb function in persons with long term paraplegia and implications for independence: Part 1. Spinal Cord. 1994; **32**(4):211-218

[23] Pentland W, Twomey l. The weight-bearing upper extremity in women with long term paraplegia. Spinal Cord. 1991; **29**(8):521-530

[24] Samuelsson K, Tropp H, Gerdle B. Shoulder pain and its consequences in paraplegic spinal cord-injured, wheelchair users. Spinal Cord. 2004; **42**(1):41-46

[25] Sie IH, Waters RL, Adkins RH, Gellman H. Upper extremity pain in the post rehabilitation spinal cord injured patient. Archives of Physical Medicine and Rehabilitation. 1992;**73**(1):44-48

[26] Subbarao JV, Klopfstein J, Turpin R. Prevalence and impact of wrist and shoulder pain in patients with spinal cord injury. The Journal of Spinal Cord Medicine. 1995;**18**(1):9-13

[27] Michael J, Krause JS, Iammertse DP. 1999. Recent trends in mortality and causes of death among persons with spinal cord injury. Archives of Physical Medicine and Rehabilitation. 1999; **80**(11):1411-1419

[28] Jackson AB, Dijkers M, Devivo MJ, Poczatek RB. A demographic profile of new traumatic spinal cord injuries: Change and stability over 30 years. Archives of Physical Medicine and Rehabilitation. 2004;**85**(11):1740-1748

[29] Degroot GJ. A few good women: Gender stereotypes, the military and peacekeeping. International Peacekeeping. 2001;**8**(2):23-38

[30] Kidd D, Stewart G, Baldry J, Johnson J, Rossiter D, Petruckevitch A, et al. The functional independence measure: A comparative validity and reliability study. Disability and Rehabilitation. 1995;**17**(1):10-14

[31] Curtis K, Roach K, Applegate E, Amar T, Benbow C, Genecco T, et al. Reliability, and validity of the wheelchair user's shoulder pain index (WUPSI). Spinal Cord. 1995;**33**(10): 595-601

[32] Mayhew TP, Rothstein JM, Finucane SD, Lamb RL. Performance characteristics of the kin-com® dynamometer. Physical Therapy. 1994; **74**(11):1047-1054

[33] Innes E. Handgrip strength testing: A review of the literature. Australian Occupational Therapy Journal. 1999; **46**(3):120-140

[34] Johnson EW, editor. Practical Electromyography (Rehabilitation Medicine Library). Hammond, IN, USA: Lippincott Williams and Wilkins; 1980

[35] Kroenke K. Studying symptoms: Sampling and measurement issues. Annals of Internal Medicine. 2001;**134**(9 part 2):844-853

[36] Stark T, Walker B, Phillips JK, Fejer R, Beck R. Hand-held dynamometry correlation with the gold standard isokinetic dynamometry: A systematic review. PM & R. 2011;**3**(5): 472-479

[37] Higgins JP, Thompson SG. Quantifying heterogeneity in a meta-analysis. Statistics in Medicine. 2002; **21**(11):1539-1558

[38] Bhandari A, Wagner T. Self-reported utilization of health care services: Improving measurement and accuracy. Medical Care Research and Review. 2006;**63**(2):217-235

[39] Short ME, Goetzel RZ, Pei X, Tabrizi MJ, Ozminkowski RJ, Gibson TB, et al. How accurate are self-reports? Analysis of self-reported health care utilization and absence when compared with administrative data. Journal of Occupational and Environmental Medicine. 2009;**51**(7):786-796

[40] Chan D. So why ask me? Are self-report data really that bad? In: Lance CE, Vandenberg RJ, editors. Statistical and Methodological Myths and Urban Legends: Doctrine, Verity and Fable in the Organizational and Social Sciences. New York: Routledge/Taylor & Francis Group; 2009. pp. 309-336

[41] Ritter PL, Stewart AL, Kaymaz H, Sobel DS, Block DA, Lorig KR. Self-reports of health care utilization compared to provider records. Journal of Clinical Epidemiology. 2001;**54**(2): 136-141

[42] Roberts RO, Bergstralh EJ, Schmidt I, Jacobsen SJ. Comparison of self-reported and medical record health care utilization measures. Journal of Clinical Epidemiology. 1996;**b49**(9):989-995

[43] Cleary PD, Jette AM. The validity of self-reported physician utilization measures. Medical Care. 1984;**22**(9): 796-803

[44] Van Den Beuken-Van Everdingen MH, De Rijke JM, Kessels AG, Schouten HC, Van Kleef M, Patijn J. Prevalence of pain in patients with cancer: A systematic review of the past 40 years. Annals of Oncology. 2007; **18**(9):1437-1449

[45] Garber MC, Uau DP, Erickson SR, Aikens JE, Lawrence JB. The concordance of self-report with other

measures of medication adherence: A summary of the literature. Medical Care. 2004;**42**(7):649-652

[46] Muhajarine N, Mustard C, Roos II, Young TK, Gelskey DE. Comparison of survey and physician claims data for detecting hypertension. Journal of Clinical Epidemiology. 1997;**50**(6): 711-718

[47] Siddall PJ, Loeser JD. Pain following spinal cord injury. Spinal Cord. 2001; **39**(2):63-73

[48] Siddall PJ, Taylor DA, Cousins MJ. Classification of pain following spinal cord injury. Spinal Cord. 1997;**35**(2):69-75

[49] Adriaansen JJ, Post MW, De Groot S, Van Asbeck FW, Stolwijk-Swüste JM, Tepper M, et al. Secondary health conditions in persons with spinal cord injury: A longitudinal study from one to five years post-discharge. Journal of Rehabilitation Medicinc. 2013;**45**(10): 1016-1022

[50] Burke D, Fullen BM, Lennon O. Pain profiles in a community dwelling population following spinal cord injury: A national survey. The Journal of Spinal Cord Medicine. 2019;**42**(2):201-211

[51] O'Connor AB. Neuropathic pain: Quality-of-life impact, costs and cost effectiveness of therapy. PharmacoEconomics. 2009;**27**(2):95-112

[52] Finnerup NB, Baastrup C. Spinal cord injury pain: Mechanisms and management. Current Pain and Headache Reports. 2012;**16**(3):207-216

[53] Nichols PJ, Norman PA, Ennis JR. 1979. Wheelchair user's shoulder? Shoulder pain in patients with spinal cord lesions. Scandinavian Journal of Rehabilitation Medicine. 1979;**11**(1): 29-32

[54] Dhssps NI. Proposals for the Reform of the Northern Ireland Wheelchair Service. Northern Ireland: DHSSPS; 2008

[55] Moffett L. A pension for injured victims of the troubles: Reparations or reifying victim hierarchy? Northern Ireland Legal Quarterly. 2016;**66**(4): 297-319

[56] Widerström-Noga E, Biering-Sørensen F, Bryce T, Cardenas DD, Finnerup NB, Jensen MP, et al. The international spinal cord injury pain basic data set. Spinal Cord. 2008;**46**(12): 818-823

[57] Widerström-Noga E, Biering-Sørensen F, Bryce T, Cardenas DD, Finnerup NB, Jensen MP, et al. The international spinal cord injury pain basic data set (version 2.0). Spinal Cord. 2014;**52**(4):282

Chapter 4

Pott's Paraplegia

Nazmin Ahmed, Md. Shahidul Islam Khan and Md. Kamrul Ahsan

Abstract

Spinal tuberculosis (TB) is a worldwide public health issue which is one of the main causes of disability. In regions with high TB incidence, Pott's disease, also known as spinal tuberculosis, is also highly prevalent. Osteoarticular tuberculosis, which affects 1–2% of people with tuberculosis, is always a secondary infection that individuals with primary TB elsewhere in the body have. The most serious kind of bone TB is Pott's paraplegia. The spinal cord is compressed, there is a gradual neurologic loss, and there may be deformity as the infection often starts from the vertebral body with noticeable damage and creation of a cold abscess. The management and treatment of spinal TB is challenging and intricate. Despite the availability of cutting-edge surgical techniques, imaging modalities, and anti-tubercular chemotherapy, managing Pott's paraplegia can be challenging, particularly for those strains having multidrug resistant capacity. In order to achieve the desired neurological outcome, therapy should be tailored to each patient's unique needs. Early diagnosis and prompt therapy are the main initial challenges in the management. The pathophysiology, imaging differential diagnosis, neuroimaging characteristics, surgical choice, and neurological prognosis of Pott's paraplegia patients from previous literatures have been highlighted in this chapter.

Keywords: Pott's paraplegia, tuberculosis, neuroimaging, surgery, disability

1. Introduction

A typical manifestation of extrapulmonary tuberculosis or osteoarticular tuberculosis is Pott disease, commonly referred to as tuberculous spondylitis. It can cause substantial functional impairment and is associated with a significant morbidity. Since ancient times, TB has been recognized and Indian medical writings from about 1000 and 600 BCE have descriptions of it. Sir Percival Pott first identified the clinical symptoms of tuberculosis of the spinal column in 1779, including kyphotic deformity and neurological deficiency in patients from Europe [1–4].

During the nineteenth and twentieth centuries, the identification of the causative pathogenic microorganism (*Mycobacterium tuberculosis*), improvements in diagnostic techniques, the development of the Bacillus Calmette-Guerin (BCG) vaccine, chemotherapeutic drugs, and surgical techniques had given humanity significantly better defense against the condition. Since the beginning of time, *M. tuberculosis* has shared the planet with birds, fish, animals, and people [1, 5].

Through the hematogenous pathway and spine, *M. tuberculosis* enters the bone, joints and for 50% of cases, spinal involvement is found. Around 90–95% of the vertebral body can have *M. tuberculosis*, and 5–10% of the posterior vertebral arch's numerous components. The radiological manifestations of anterior spinal TB are so well-known that plane radiographs are the primary tool used to diagnose the majority of cases. Additional helpful tools include imaging techniques like computed tomography (CT scan) and magnetic resonance imaging (MRI) [6–10].

Due to international migration, particularly among the immunosuppressed population, the Pott's illness has lately exhibited a substantial resurgence in industrialized countries. The global community has faced a significant difficulty as a result. Over the past few decades, there has been a concerning rise in the incidence of multidrug-resistant bacterial strains of TB in underdeveloped countries. These factors explain why the illness is still a serious threat to global public health [11–14].

1.1 Epidemiology

Pott's illness is particularly prevalent in nations with high rates of TB and HIV/AIDS, but a firm diagnosis is still challenging to make. Osteoarticular tuberculosis, which affects 1–2% of people with the disease, is always a secondary infection that individuals with primary TB elsewhere in the body have. In the vast majority of instances (80%), it may be challenging to identify the illness's initial location, although the sickness is always present. Osteoarticular tuberculosis is a localized symptom of a disease that affects the entire body [1–4, 15].

The microorganism *M. tuberculosis* is mostly found in the lung and causes TB in around one-third of the world's population. Recently, the World Health Organization's (WHO) reported the global prevalence and mortality rates of TB based on the data of 200 countries, which indicates a decrease of prevalence since 1990, suggesting significant progress of TB control. According to a previous conducted study of 2013, between 1990 and 2010, TB-related fatalities has been reduced by almost 40% [16–18]. Despite significant attempts to prevent TB infection, there have been recent increases of TB cases immigration from endemic areas to non-endemic regions of the world. The increase of poverty, unemployment, AIDS infections, and resistance to anti-TB chemotherapeutic medicines also made the TB control measures challenging [16, 17].

1.2 Pathogenesis

The most frequent cause of TB in humans is *M. tuberculosis. Mycobacterium microti, Mycobacterium bovis,* and *Mycobacterium africanum* are other mycobacteria that cause human TB. *Mycobacterium* is a meticulous, aerobic bacteria that grows slowly. *Mycobacterium*-containing droplets travel through the air and land on the lungs, where alveolar macrophages consume them. Most of these microorganisms are eliminated. Few are capable of surviving and proliferating in macrophages, which causes a type IV inflammatory response that causes granulomas to develop. In this granuloma, bacteria can remain latent and persist for decades [19].

Whether an infection is managed or not depends on how well the host cell-mediated immune response functions. *Mycobacterium* may escape from granuloma if the immune response against the pathogen is insufficient. A *mycobacterium* that has escaped can either cause an active lung infection or it can enter other organs through hematogenous and lymphatic routes. With hematogenous spread of infection from a primary location, spinal involvement is typically subsequent. Spinal involvement originates from the lungs or the genitourinary system [20, 21].

Since the intervertebral disc lacks a blood supply of its own, the infection travels there from the vertebra next to it. Mycobacterium enters the highly vascular cancellous bone of the vertebral body through the venous or arterial pathway. Paradisal involvement results from the transmission of infection through the vascular plexus formed by the arterial arcade produced from the posterior and anterior arteries. The valveless Batson's paravertebral venous plexus system allows for a free flow of blood which is dependent on pressure [22–24].

1.3 Clinical features

There are several early signs of tuberculosis include night sweats, fever, weight loss etc. whereas, spread to the spine would be determined by a severe back pain, this Patients may face difficulty in standing and walk. Severe back pain is the most frequent symptom of Pott's disease, however, systematic symptoms such as anorexia, fever, fatigue, night sweats, weight loss etc. are also common. The swelling of infection site might cause weakness or numbness in legs. In complicated tubercular spine disease patient may present with rest pain, deformity, bone destruction, instability and sometimes radicular pain would be main symptom. In Pott's paraplegia, presence of neurologic deficit is not quite common and percentage of incidence greatly varies (5–100%) due to stages of disease. Pott's illness can therefore result in a significant curvature of the spine and limb paralysis. Spinal cord involvement in Pott's illness can be caused by direct pressure from abscess development and/or bone sequestrum [25–27].

1.4 Neuroimaging features

The majority of tuberculomas were numerous and dispersed across the cerebral hemispheres. Additional spinal cord imaging may be helpful in determining the entire degree of the illness in patients with quadriparesis or paraparesis. Worse prognosis is linked to spinal cord involvement and it is clear that CNS TB is complex. Studies has identified some difference between baseline scans and follow-up scans for majority of cases though only for less than 5% of patients second follow-up scan performed. These follow-up scans usually performed within 3 months of primary scans. After 3 months, we could presume the stabilization of disease process, which is why patients did not get follow-up scans later period such as after 6 month or annually. On subsequent scans, the size and number of tuberculomas either stayed the same, changed, or rose or decreased [28–31].

According to previous studies, cerebral infarction is an independent predictor of poor prognosis of CNS TB those are mostly acute in nature. On subsequent imaging, several patients had additional infarcts form. There are also some contradictions regarding the infarction's location. Therefore, in the future, it's important to strive for a varied and extensive TB distribution in research and intervention studies. In order to connect the site of the infarction with a worse outcome, some studies suggested CT scans in a pediatric population [32, 33].

1.5 Progressive neurological deficit in Pott's paraplegia

During the active Pott's paraplegia stage of or after recovery there might be some neurological deficit. The vertebral collapse due to TB would result in the involvement of anterior spinal tract. Later, the posterior column deficiency is followed by a gradual involvement of the lateral spinal pathways. Scores such as Frankel and ASIA ratings would also be used to categorize the neurological deficit in spinal tuberculosis. The most helpful classification for Pott paraplegia with spinal cord involvement is the modified version of Tuli classification [34–38]. Motor fibers are crushed initially because they are not located similarly, as seen in the typical Pott's paraplegia or anterior spinal TB. As a result, the sensory fibers are only implicated later [39–42].

When compression occurs due to anterior or posterior spinal tuberculosis, pressure is initially applied to the column of cerebrospinal fluid around the cord before being conveyed to the ligamentum denticulatum. The claims made by Bosworth et al. that the tubercular pus contains a chemical that prevents the spinal cord from conducting properly appear speculative. The classification of Pott's disease, whether brought on by anterior or posterior spinal TB, should primarily be based on the level of motor involvement to represent the severity of cord compression. As the degree of compression rises, sensory and autonomic functional loss is increased. Sensory recovery comes before the motor recovery (**Figure 1**) [34, 43].

A previous study has documented 100 instances of TB spine with neurological consequences and among them 33% were reported before 4 weeks, majority (40%) were after 4 weeks and within 3 months, and remaining 27% after 3 months of the neurological deficit first appeared. When an intraspinal tuberculous granuloma is initially observed, it frequently exhibits compressive myelopathy or a cauda equina lesion with sphincter involvement. They are diagnosed with "spinal tumor syndrome," which covers both tumorous and non-tumorous disorders of the spinal cord and meninges, because they exhibit no clinical spinal deformity upon inspection [44–46].

1.6 Diagnostic studies

Mycobacterium culture is the gold standard for diagnosing tuberculosis, however as it's a fastidious microorganism relying solely on positive cultures for diagnosis might

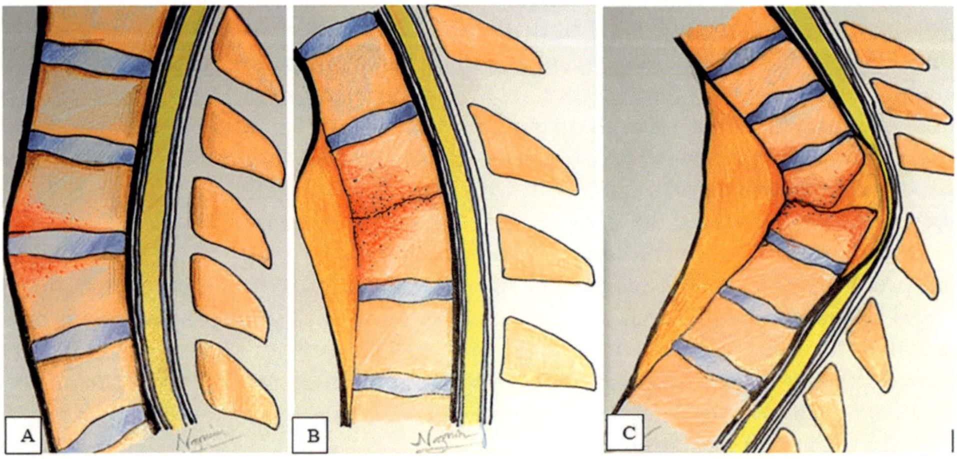

Figure 1.
Schematic picture demonstrates the pattern of involvement of musculoskeletal and soft tissue structures in Pott's disease leads to progressive paraplegia; (A) showing only paradiscal VB involvement with preservation of the disc, vertebral arch and no compression on spinal cord; (B) showing paradiscal VB involvement as well as intervertebral disc with formation of abscess by stripping the ALL and (C) demonstrates huge epidural abscess which is responsible for significant compression on spinal cord with local kyphotic deformity. At this stage, patient develops paraparesis followed by paraplegia.

have low sensitivity. To confirm the diagnosis, further laboratory reference standards such as microbiological, immunological, hematological, serological, and other diagnostic resources should be employed. MRI is most frequently used for the diagnosis and cold abscess by using ultrasound. Myelography's has important role diagnosis of patients who do not recover neurologically and in situations where there are multiple skipped multifocal spinal lesions to identify which lesion is causing compression [47–49].

2. Imaging modalities

2.1 Radiography

With a 15% sensitivity, plain radiographs were proposed previously as an imaging modality for Pott's disease. As a first stage diagnosis process, conventional lateral radiographs are used to look for TB infection. These radiographs typically show osteolysis affecting the entire vertebral body with diffuse osteopenia [7, 50–52].

2.2 Computed tomography (CT) scan

With great sensitivity, computed tomography (CT) can assist in the diagnosis at a far earlier stage than ordinary x-rays (100%). CT is a valuable and common diagnostic tool, in cases with Pott's disease which would able to demonstrates the extension of soft tissue involvement clearly. For the purpose of making a diagnosis, CT scans can also help in image-guided biopsy [7, 50–53].

2.3 Magnetic resonance imaging (MRI)

With a 100% sensitivity and an 80% specificity, magnetic resonance imaging (MRI) is the most helpful modality in the diagnosis of spinal TB. The location of the abscess, the degree of soft tissue enhancement, and spinal canal impairment are all best detected with MRI. MRI with gadolinium enhancement might offer more details on the diagnosis. We can also identify non-contiguous vertebral involvement by doing screening sequences that include the whole spine. MRI can be used to evaluate therapy response [54–56]. MRI can also demonstrate the number of lesion and their locations in cold abscesses. Recently published report demonstrates that the early detection of inflammatory oedema could be ensured by T2 STIR images [16].

2.4 Nuclear imaging

Nuclear imaging can provide descriptive evidences of the activities in the affected tissues. These techniques are unable to assist distinguish between cancer or other pyogenic diseases and tubercular infections [57].

2.5 Laboratory tests

Laboratory test such as Erythrocyte sedimentation rate (ESR) and C-reactive protein (CRP) are less common test. ESR has a sensitivity of 90% and CRP a sensitivity of 71%, however has more specificity than ESR [58]. The serological tests have a round of limitations. IgG and IgM (antibody test) levels is not effective to determine the difference of natural TB infection, vaccinated person, active disease, or healed person [59, 60]. Traditional TB culture, Acid-fast bacilli staining, BACTEC assay are some common laboratory techniques [61]. Isolation of *Mycobacterium tuberculosis* with a computed tomography (CT)-guided needle biopsy or open surgical intervention can yield an accurate diagnosis. In cases receiving anti-TB chemotherapy in the lead up to surgery, it is difficult to show typical acid-fast bacilli on staining with hematoxylin-eosin, and results of TB cultures are typically negative in such cases. Histological examination of formalin-fixed and paraffin-embedded tissue specimen blocks typically provides granulomatous pattern with caseating necrosis and giant-cell granuloma [25, 26, 62].

2.6 Molecular diagnosis

Various types of molecular techniques are useful for the diagnosis with high sensitivity and specificity. Polymerase chain reaction (PCR) with a sensitivity of 75% and specificity of 97%) is used in paucibacillary, extrapulmonary TB infections. Fully automated Gene Xpert MTB/RIF help in the diagnosis of resistance towards antibiotics with high sensitivity and specificity [12, 63]. In between 72% and 97% of patients, specific features such Langhans large cells, epithelioid cell granuloma, and caseating necrosis can be detected through histopathological examinations [64, 65].

2.7 Tests to detect latent tuberculosis

The skin hypersensitivity test has been advocated as a low-cost test; however, it is not a reliable test in areas where patients are immunocompromised. Some studies also suggest the use of the enzyme-linked immunosorbent test (ELISA) and the interferon-gamma release assay [66, 67].

3. Treatment of Pott's paraplegia

Before treatment of Pott's paraplegia, it is important determine the severity of the spinal TB disease, based on presentation and symptoms. Uncomplicated disease is treated with antitubercular treatment (chemotherapy) and complicated cases usually need surgical intervention with chemotherapy [68].

The most helpful classification for Pott paraplegia with spinal cord involvement is the modified version of Tuli's classification which consist of five stages. The First stage includes intense tendon reflexes, ankle clonus, plantar or Babinski extensor. During the second stage patient face a motor deficit (UMN-type) with spasticity. In the stage three patient become spastic and bedridden (motor crore: around 0–30). Patient become bedridden including a severe sensory deficit/pressure sores in the 4th stage. The final or 5th stage is similar to 4th stage bladder or bowel involvement [34, 35].

Oguz et al. proposed a new classification system for Pott's disease named Gulhane Askeri Tıp Akademisi widely known as GATA. Where they divided Pott's Paraplegia based on clinical and radiological status into three categories (IA/B, II, and III). GATA suggested surgical treatment for patients with Type IB (no neurological deficit), Type II and Type III (with or without neurological deficit). M. Turgut et al. (2017) presented we a new simple modified classification system from GATA system. The modified system is a simple guide for treatment planning in patients with Pott's disease for young spinal surgeons [69, 70].

3.1 Conservative treatment and chemotherapy

The cornerstones in the treatment of spinal TB are antitubercular medications (Isoniazid, Rifampicin, Ethambutol, and Pyrazinamide). It addresses both the main tubercular foci present elsewhere in the body as well as the spinal TB. Also recommended is higher-dose, shorter-course intermittent chemotherapy that is administered three times each week [71].

Recently established protocols recommends anti-TB chemotherapy with 2 months of isoniazid (INH) (5–15 mg/kg), pyrazinamide (PZA) (30–40 mg/kg), rifampicin (RIF) (10–20 mg/kg), and ethambutol (EMB) (15–25 mg/kg), followed by INH and RIF (next 4 months) [16]. According to the British Medical Research Council, combined chemotherapy should be used to treat tuberculous spondylitis of the thoracolumbar spine for 6–9 months. A 4.5-month ultra-short course of chemotherapy has been suggested, although bigger trials and longer follow-up studies are still needed [71].

In addition to latent and quickly growing forms, tubercle bacilli can also exist in intracellular and extracellular forms. In order to combat the bacilli in their many phases or forms and decrease the occurrence of medication resistance, a multi-drug therapy is required. The WHO advises a six-month course of multidrug anti-tubercular therapy, which includes 2 months of "initiation" phase therapy with a four/five-drug regimen and 4 months of "continuation" phase therapy with a two-drug regimen containing isoniazid and rifampicin. The American thoracic spine society (ATSS) advises a 9-month therapy plan using the same medications. When there is resistance to or poor tolerance to first-line treatments, additional second-line anti-tubercular therapies, such as kanamycin, capreomycin, pyrazinamide, and amikacin, among others, are often recommended. Beside some contradiction, the WHO has continued to recommend DOTS therapy for optimum results [72–75].

Research conducted in in the pre-chemotherapeutic period observed that, up to 66% of patients with Pott's paraplegia demonstrated neurological improvement by strictly conservative therapy. The idea was bolstered in the post-chemotherapeutic period by the observation that pure conservative treatment with chemotherapy resulted in neurological improvement in 60–80%of patients [47, 76–79].

4. Surgical management

4.1 Principles

The phrase "middle route regimen" was first used in the context of treating TB by *Tuli et al.* This protocol suggested medical management for all patients together with surgical management when it was necessary, such as in cases of chemotherapy failure, neurological weakness, recurrent illness, instability, neuro deficiency, incapacitating pain, or deformity. Because tubercle bacilli do not create a biofilm, implants can be used to stabilize tubercular infections [12, 80–82].

Neurosurgeons and orthopedic surgeons that specialize in spine surgery usually treat Pott's paraplegia. In individuals with Pott's illness who have signs of spinal cord or nerve root compression, researchers advise surgical decompression in addition to medicinal care. In order to achieve decompression in individuals with spinal instability, percutaneous needle aspiration of the caseous necrosis has been recommended. Due to the severe state of the disease in the majority of patients, a meta-analysis recommended treating the condition with anti-TB chemotherapy and surgery. For high-risk Pott's disease patients, minimally invasive interventional radiology procedures, open or percutaneous internal fixation techniques, and anti-TB chemotherapy have recently been introduced [16, 25, 26, 83, 84].

4.2 Anterior approach, posterior approach and combined approach

Debridement using an anterior approach have historically been employed to treat the diseased tissues directly since TB spine mostly affects the anterior spinal components. However, the anterior approach has reportedly been linked to significant side effects, including death, graft-related problems, and method-related issues. Patients without any involvement of the posterior spinal structures, without panvertebral illness, are the best candidates for anterior surgery [85–87].

For a variety of reasons, including ease of use and familiarity, posterior techniques are more frequently used in contemporary spine surgery for TB spondylitis. The advantage include, less morbidity, strong pedicle screw system, and the capacity for circumferential decompression [88–92].

As the combination method is usually linked with major morbidities and problems, it should only be used for severe destructive lesions with severe deformities or fundamentally unstable spines. The methods might be applied in a single stage or many stages [93, 94]. Based on the aforementioned reasons, majority of surgeons propose combined anterior and posterior operation which enables sufficient focus debridement and stabilization after kyphosis correction (**Figure 2**) [95–97].

4.3 Surgery in healed tuberculosis

Age, the degree of the deformity, concomitant conditions, the region of the spine involved, the number of levels involved, and the surgeon's choice should all be taken into account before deciding whether to operate on a patient with an unstable illness. In the thoracic and thoracolumbar levels at the peak of kyphosis, anterior approach might be particularly challenging. The most common posterior techniques are closing opening wedge osteotomy, pedicle subtraction osteotomy/closing wedge osteotomy, posterior vertebral column resection, transpedicular decancellation, and Ponte's osteotomy. In more severe abnormalities, diseases affecting two or three vertebrae, or complicated revision procedures, both anterior and posterior techniques may be necessary [98–102].

4.4 Management during pregnancy

Pott's disease during pregnancy reported to be rare & can be associated with destruction of the intervertebral disc & adjacent vertebrae that can lead to cord compression. The effects of extrapulmonary tuberculosis infection during pregnancy depend on the site of involvement, the severity and duration of disease, and the occurrence of pregnancy-related complications. The safety of the first-line drugs for the management of active tuberculosis in pregnancy has been established, and therapy improves both maternal and neonatal outcomes. There is no malformation or teratogenicity identified in pregnant patients taking these drugs. Streptomycin should be avoided in pregnancy as it is ototoxic to the fetus. The WHO recommends ATT for 9 months but most experts prefer to continue ATT for one to 2 years. Some experts advocate early surgical decompression in all while others prefer to operate after delivery [103–105].

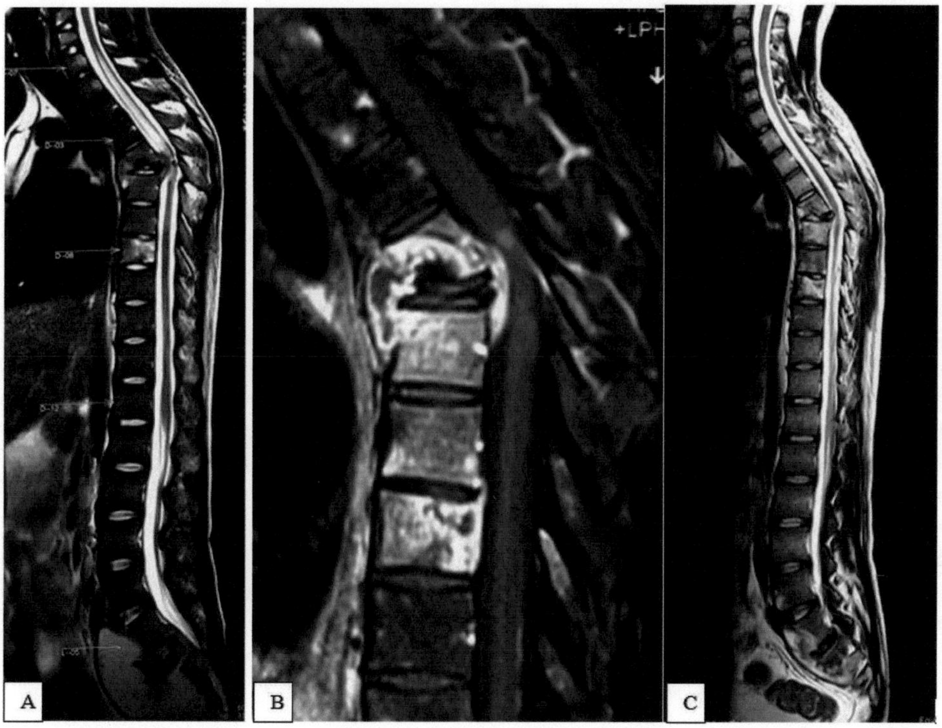

Figure 2.
A 23-year-old male presented with progressive spastic paraparesis for 2 months with intact autonomic function. MRI, midsagittal T2WI-whole spine screening film demonstrated hyperintense signal change sporadically involved the spinal column. Variable stages of VB and disc involvement, prevertebral and epidural abscess formation, kyphotic deformity, significant spinal cord compression and proximal syrinx formation present (A). After administration of gadolinium, there is heterogenous contrast enhancement (B). Patient underwent percuatenous drainage of the presacral abscess and received antitubercular chemotherapy, follow up MRI after 1 month demonstrated resolution of the syrinx, improvement of abnormal signal changes, as well as extent of spinal cord compression and (C). Later on, decompression and fixation done on D3,4,6,7 in second sitting to decompress the spinal cord and to correct the deformity.

As per general guidelines for spinal surgery in pregnant women with progressive neurological deficit, delivery should be induced or cesarean section is performed before spinal surgery at 34–36 weeks of gestation or later. In cases earlier than 34–36 weeks of gestation, prepartum spinal surgery should be performed. Surgery and anesthesia during advanced pregnancy are associated with increased risk of spontaneous abortion, preterm labor, prematurity and low birth weight. Pregnant women with paraplegia have increased incidence of urinary tract infection, decubitus ulcer, preterm labour & autonomic hyperflexia [104–106].

4.5 Management of children

Children are one of the most vulnerable group for being affected by the Pott's paraplegia. Hematogenous spread from the original site of infection is the major method of infection in children. Children with spinal TB frequently experience symptoms in the dorsal spine; only around 5% of kids experience symptoms in the cervical spine [107–110].

The mainstay of the care of pediatric spinal TB continues to be conservative therapy, which includes chemotherapy and orthopedic immobilization. The American

Thoracic Society and the Centers for Disease Control and Prevention made it obvious that a minimum of 12 months of treatment is necessary for bone and joint TB. However, some recent findings claimed that a shorter duration would be suitable for those with spinal TB [111–113].

Large abscesses, especially those in the psoas muscle, should be treated surgically. In addition, children who exhibit or acquire neurological deficiency during follow-up must have surgery to stop permanent paralysis or deteriorating deformities. In children with spinal TB, a severe kyphosis of more than 60° occurs in around 3 percent of cases. Children under the age of 10, the involvement of three or more vertebral bodies, and the location of the lesion in the thoracic spine are risk factors for severe kyphotic deformity. A severe kyphosis compromises one's appearance and causes cardiac malfunction and compression of the spinal cord. The surgical method is also not uniform globally. To describe the surgical method, processes, surgical stages, challenges, and difficulties for correcting the kyphosis of 60° or more, prospective studies are required [111, 114, 115]. One-stage posterior instrumentation combined anterior debridement and fusion were demonstrated to be a safe and effective method to achieve spinal decompression and kyphosis correction in children with thoracic and lumbar spinal TB.

In treatment of children with multiple-level tuberculosis causing evident kyphosis and with extensive abscesses, posterior screw instrumentation prior to anterior approach usually applied. Posterior instrumentation enabled best correction of the sagittal profile, restoration of vertebral height and reconstruction of segmental stability by appropriate distraction in active stages of spinal TB. Ponte osteotomies usually performed to increase flexibility and facilitate correction. For patients with seriously compressed spinal cord, laminectomy is performed before deformity correction. Furthermore, combined anterior and posterior fusions can prevent the imbalanced spinal growth of children, and maintain long-term correction [116, 117].

4.6 Rest, braces and traction

Braces have importance and are still frequently required. Forcing people to slumber for more than 6–9 months on a hard bed or a plaster-of-Paris bed may even be detrimental, leading to skin, lung, gastrointestinal, and metabolic issues. Braces are frequently more torment and pseudo-satisfaction tools than actual tools. Due to the significant deforming pressures, braces cannot stop the progression of kyphotic deformity. Therefore, braces are typically not very helpful. Any brace that a patient often removes for personal care, a bath, or pain loses its intended function. The only brace which may be useful is trauma cervical brace for cranio-occipital and few cases of cervical spine tuberculosis. Halo frames are used for stabilization, not for traction or distraction [71, 118].

4.7 Future research on Pott's Paraplegia

During the last two decade a significant improvement has been made in terms of diagnosis and treatment of Pott's Paraplegia. However, more research is required regarding the improvement management and treatment especially surgical procedure in various conditions. Research is required for development of more prompt diagnosis, management and treatment to reduce severe consequences and complications. Extensive study is required on the preventive treatment and quick screening of Pott's disease among children. Now a days, MDR is bothering all countries as it requires more investigations for proper treatments. Early identification of drug resistance and prescription of suitable drugs for appropriate duration is the key to manage Pott's spine. We also recommend more research in the area rehabilitation as it is a crucial component to improve the quality of life of patients. There is also a lack of research in the area of kyphosis correction.

5. Conclusion

The treatment of spinal TB illness is difficult and intricate. Spinal tuberculosis can be treated by anybody who can cure TB. The contributions of all levels of health service provider are highly important for the management of Pott's paraplegia, even though the treating surgeon plays the majority of the patient management role. When there is a neurological deficiency or deformity, orthopedic surgeons are typically needed. With very few exceptions, managing Pott's spine and paraplegia based on paraplegia grading is straightforward, rational, effective, and simple to remember. Early diagnosis and prompt therapy are the main initial challenges in the management of the condition. The next significant step is determining the disease-related consequences and making the right choice regarding whether long-term treatment is necessary in addition to surgical procedures. The difficulties in administering long-term chemotherapy, such as side effects and complications from the medication, problems with compliance, socioeconomic variables, and others, are also very important.

Author details

Nazmin Ahmed[1*], Md. Shahidul Islam Khan[2] and Md. Kamrul Ahsan[2]

1 Department of Neurosurgery, Ibrahim Cardiac Hospital and Research Institute (A Centre for Cardiovascular, Neuroscience and Organ Transplant Units), Dhaka, Bangladesh

2 Spine Surgery Unit, Department of Orthopaedic Surgery, Bangabandhu Sheikh Mujib Medical University, Dhaka, Bangladesh

*Address all correspondence to: nazmin.bsmmu@gmail.com

References

[1] Taylor GM, Murphy E, Hopkins R, Rutland P, Chistov Y. First report of mycobacterium bovis DNA in human remains from the iron age. Microbiology. 2007;**153**(4):1243-1249

[2] Parquet RA. Percivall pott. Acta Gastroenterologica Latinoamericana. 2015;**45**(3):186-187

[3] Tuli SM. Historical aspects of Pott's disease (spinal tuberculosis) management. European Spine Journal. 2013;**22**(Suppl.4):529-538

[4] Dobson J. Percivall Pott. Annals of the Royal College of Surgeons of England. 1972;**50**(1):54-65

[5] Toida I. Development of the Mycobacterium bovis BCG vaccine: Review of the historical and biochemical evidence for a genealogical tree. Tubercle and Lung Disease. 2000;**80**(6):291

[6] Kumar K. Spinal tuberculosis, natural history of disease, classifications and principles of management with historical perspective. European Journal of Orthopaedic Surgery and Traumatology. 2016;**26**(6):551-558

[7] Desai SS. Early diagnosis of spinal tuberculosis by MRI. Journal of Bone and Joint Surgery - Series B. 1994;**76**(6):863-869. Available from: http://www.embase.com/search/results?subaction=viewrecord&from=export&id=L24368436

[8] Jain R, Sawhney S, Berry M. Computer tomography of vertebral tuberculosis: Patterns of bone destruction. Clinical Radiology. 1993;**47**(3):196-199

[9] Hoffman EB, Crosier JH, Cremin BJ. Imaging in children with spinal tuberculosis. A comparison of radiography, computed tomography and magnetic resonance imaging. Journal of Bone and Joint Surgery - Series B. 1993;**75**(2):233-239

[10] Chongchitnant P. Computed tomography of spinal tuberculosis. Journal of the Medical Association of Thailand. 1992;**75**(10):560-564

[11] Shetty AP, Viswanathan VK, Kanna RM, Shanmuganathan R. Tubercular spondylodiscitis in elderly is a more severe disease: A report of 66 consecutive patients. European Spine Journal. 2017;**26**(12):3178-3186

[12] Rajasekaran S, Soundararajan DCR, Shetty AP, Kanna RM. Spinal tuberculosis: Current concepts. Glob The Spine Journal. 2018;**8**(4_suppl):96S-108S

[13] Arockiaraj J, Karthik R, Michael JS, Amritanand R, David KS, Krishnan V, et al. "Need of the hour": Early diagnosis and management of multidrug resistant tuberculosis of the spine: An analysis of 30 patients from a 'high multidrug resistant tuberculosis burden' country. Asian Spine Journal. 2019;**13**(2):265-271

[14] McLain RF, Isada C. Spinal tuberculosis deserves a place on the radar screen. Cleveland Clinic Journal of Medicine. 2004;**71**(7):537-549

[15] Simonton DK. Creativity in the later years: Optimistic prospects for achievement. The Gerontologist. 1990;**30**(5):626-631

[16] Varatharajah S, Charles YP, Buy X, Walter A, Steib JP. Update on the surgical management of Pott's disease. Orthopaedics & Traumatology, Surgery & Research. 2014;**100**(2):233-239. DOI: 10.1016/j.otsr.2013.09.013. Available

from: http://www.embase.com/search/results?subaction=viewrecord&from=export&id=L372650968%0A

[17] Dara M, Dadu A, Kremer K, Zaleskis R, Kluge HHP. Epidemiology of tuberculosis in WHO European Region and public health response. European Spine Journal. 2013;**22**(Suppl. 4):549-555

[18] WHO. Global Tuberculosis Report 2015. In: World Heal Organ. 20th ed. 2015. Available from: http://apps.who.int/iris/bitstream/10665/191102/1/9789241565059_eng.pdf

[19] Kumar V, Neradi D, Sherry B, Gaurav A, Dhatt SS. Tuberculosis of the spine and drug resistance: A review article. Neurosurgical Review. 2022;**45**(1):217-229

[20] Smith I. Mycobacterium tuberculosis pathogenesis and molecular determinants of virulence. Clinical Microbiology Reviews. 2003;**16**(3):463-496

[21] Schirmer P, Renault CA, Holodniy M. Is spinaltuberculosiscontagious?International Journal of Infectious Diseases. 2010;**14**(8):e659-e666

[22] Ansari S, Amanullah M, Ahmad K, Rauniyar RK. Pott's spine: Diagnostic imaging modalities and technology advancements. North American Journal of Medical Sciences. 2013;**5**(7):404-411

[23] Gautam MP, Karki P, Rijal S, Singh R. Pott's spine and paraplegia. Journal of Nepal Medical Association. 2005;**44**(159):106-115

[24] Tuli S. Tuberculosis of the Skeletal System. Tuberculosis of the Skeletal System. 2004;**3**(6):103-109

[25] Turgut M. Spinal tuberculosis (Pott's disease): Its clinical presentation, surgical management, and outcome. A survey study on 694 patients. Neurosurgical Review. 2001;**24**(1):8-13

[26] Turgut M. Multifocal extensive spinal tuberculosis (Pott's disease) involving cervical, thoracic and lumbar vertebrae. British Journal of Neurosurgery. 2001;**15**(2):142-146. DOI: 10.1080/02688690120036856. Available from: http://www.embase.com/search/results?subaction=viewrecord&from=export&id=L32423266%0A

[27] Rezai AR, Lee M, Cooper PR, Errico TJ, Koslow M. Modern management of spinal tuberculosis. Neurosurgery. 1995;**36**(1):87-98

[28] Azeemuddin M, Alvi A, Sayani R, Khan MK, Farooq S, Beg MA, et al. Neuroimaging findings in tuberculosis: A single-center experience in 559 cases. Journal of Neuroimaging. 2019;**29**(5):657-668

[29] Sonmez G, Ozturk E, Sildiroglu HO, Mutlu H, Cuce F, Senol MG, et al. MRI findings of intracranial tuberculomas. Clinical Imaging. 2008;**32**(2):88-92

[30] Anuradha HK, Garg RK, Sinha MK, Agarwal A, Verma R, Singh MK, et al. Intracranial tuberculomas in patients with tuberculous meningitis: Predictors and prognostic significance. The International Journal of Tuberculosis and Lung Disease. 2011;**15**(2):234-239

[31] Sheu JJ, Chiou HY, Kang JH, Chen YH, Lin HC. Tuberculosis and the risk of ischemic stroke: A 3-year follow-up study. Stroke. 2010;**41**(2):244-249

[32] Nair PP, Kalita J, Kumar S, Misra UK. MRI pattern of infarcts in basal ganglia region in patients with tuberculous meningitis. Neuroradiology. 2009;**51**(4):221-225

[33] Andronikou S, Wilmshurst J, Hatherill M, VanToorn R. Distribution

of brain infarction in children with tuberculous meningitis and correlation with outcome score at 6 months. Pediatric Radiology. 2006;**36**(12):1289-1294

[34] Jain AK, Kumar J. Tuberculosis of spine: Neurological deficit. European Spine Journal. 2013;**22**(Suppl. 4):624-633

[35] Jain AK, Sinha S. Evaluation of systems of grading of neurological deficit in tuberculosis of spine. Spinal Cord. 2005;**43**(6):375-380

[36] Frankel HL, Hancock DO, Hyslop G, Melzak J, Michaelis LS, Ungar GH, et al. The value of postural reduction in the initial management of closed injuries of the spine with paraplegia and tetraplegia. Paraplegia. 1969;**7**(3):179-192

[37] Subramani S, Shetty AP, Kanna RM, Shanmuganathan R. Ossified ligamentum flavum causing neurological deficit above the level of post-tuberculous kyphotic deformity. Journal of Clinical Orthopaedics and Trauma. 2017;**8**(2):174-177

[38] Hodgson AR, Skinsnes OK, Leong CY. The pathogenesis of Pott's paraplegia. The Journal of Bone and Joint Surgery. American Volume. 1967;**49**(6):1147-1156

[39] Kumar K. Grading of Pott's paraplegia. Journal of Neurological and Orthopaedic Medicine and Surgery. 1991;**12**(2):112-115

[40] Kumar K. Tuberculosis of spine (natural history of disease and its judicious management). Journal of the Western Pacific Orthopaedic Association. 1988;**25**(1):1-8

[41] Kumar K. A clinical study and classification of posterior spinal tuberculosis. International Orthopaedics. 1985;**9**(3):147-152

[42] Bonnin JG. Girdlestone's tuberculosis of bone and joint. BMJ. 1965;**2**:1045-1045

[43] Bosworth DM, Della Pietra A, Rahilly G. Paraplegia resulting from tuberculosis of the spine. The Journal of Bone and Joint Surgery. American Volume. 1953;**35-A**(3):735-740

[44] Babhulkar SS, Tayade WB, Babhulkar SK. Atypical spinal tuberculosis. Journal of Bone and Joint Surgery - Series B. 1984;**66**(2):239-242

[45] Teg G. Hospital B. Intraspinal tubercular granuloma. 7(3):182-185

[46] Tuli SM. Treatment of neurological complications in tuberculosis of the spine. The Journal of Bone and Joint Surgery. American Volume. 1969;**51**(4):680-692

[47] Hu S, Guo J, Ji T, Shen G, Kuang A. Multifocal osteoarticular tuberculosis of the extremities in an immunocompetent young man without pulmonary disease: A case report. Experimental and Therapeutic Medicine. 2015;**9**(6):2099-2302

[48] Kumar K, Francis AE. Myelography in Pott's paraplegia. Journal of Neurological and Orthopaedic Medicine and Surgery. 1989;**10**(2):147-150

[49] Weaver P, Lifeso RM. The radiological diagnosis of tuberculosis of the adult spine. Skeletal Radiology. 1984;**12**(3):178-186

[50] Dharmalingam M. Tuberculosis of the spine - The Sabah experience. Epidemiology, treatment and results. Tuberculosis. 2004;**84**(1-2):24-28

[51] Sinan T, Al-Khawari H, Ismail M, Ben-Nakhi A, Sheikh M. Spinal tuberculosis: CT and MRI features. Annals of Saudi Medicine. 2004;**24**(6):437-441

[52] Adapon BD, Legada BD, Lim EVA, Silao JV, Dalmacio-Cruz A. CT-guided closed biopsy of the spine. Journal of Computer Assisted Tomography. 1981;**5**(1):73-78

[53] Harisinghani MG, McLoud TC, Shepard JAO, Ko JP, Shroff MM, Mueller PR. Tuberculosis from head to toe. Radiographics. 2000;**20**(2):449-470

[54] Gouliamos AD, Kehagias DT, Lahanis S, Athanassopoulou AA, Moulopoulou ES, Kalovidouris AA, et al. MR imaging tuberculous vertebral osteomyelitis: Pictorial review. European Radiology. 2001;**11**(4):575-579

[55] Kaila R, Malhi AM, Mahmood B, Saifuddin A. The incidence of multiple level noncontiguous vertebral tuberculosis detected using whole spine MRI. Journal of Spinal Disorders & Techniques. 2007;**20**(1):78-81. DOI: 10.1097/01.bsd.0000211250.82823.0f. Available from: http://www.embase.com/search/results?subaction=viewrecord&from=export&id=L46220330%0A

[56] Kim NH, Lee HM, Suh JS. Magnetic resonance imaging for the diagnosis of tuberculous spondylitis. Spine (Phila Pa 1976). 1994;**19**(21):2451-2455

[57] Vorster M, Sathekge MM, Bomanji J. Advances in imaging of tuberculosis: The role of 18F-FDG PET and PET/CT. Current Opinion in Pulmonary Medicine. 2014;**20**(3):287-293

[58] Guo LX, Ma YZ, Li HW, Bin XH, Peng W, Luo XB. Variety of ESR and C-reactive protein levels during perioperative period in spinal tuberculosis. Zhongguo Gu Shang. 2010;**23**(3):200-202

[59] Chen CH, Chen YM, Lee CW, Chang YJ, Cheng CY, Hung JK. Early diagnosis of spinal tuberculosis. Journal of the Formosan Medical Association. 2016;**115**(10):825-836

[60] Jain AK, Jena SK, Singh MP, Dhammi IK, Ramachadran VG, Dev G. Evaluation of clinico-radiological, bacteriological, serological, molecular and histological diagnosis of osteoarticular tuberculosis. Indian Journal of Orthopaedics. 2008;**42**(2):173-177

[61] Cruciani M, Scarparo C, Malena M, Bosco O, Serpelloni G, Mengoli C. Meta-analysis of BACTEC MGIT 960 and BACTEC 460 TB, with or without Solid Media, for detection of Mycobacteria. Journal of Clinical Microbiology. 2004;**42**(5):2321-2325

[62] Sarmiento OL, Weigle KA, Alexander J, Weber DJ, Miller WC. Assessment by meta-analysis of PCR for diagnosis of smear-negative pulmonary tuberculosis. Journal of Clinical Microbiology. 2003;**41**(7):3233-3240

[63] Maynard-Smith L, Larke N, Peters JA, Lawn SD. Diagnostic accuracy of the Xpert MTB/RIF assay for extrapulmonary and pulmonary tuberculosis when testing non-respiratory samples: A systematic review. BMC Infectious Diseases. 2014;**14**(1)

[64] Alothman A, Memish ZA, Awada A, Al Mahmood S, Al Sadoon S, Rahman MM, et al. Tuberculous spondylitis analysis of 69 cases from Saudi Arabia. Spine (Phila Pa 1976). 2001;**26**(24):570-E565

[65] Johnston RA. Tuberculous spondylitis in adults. British Journal of Neurosurgery. 1989;**3**(3):417-421

[66] Brodie D, Lederer DJ, Gallardo JS, Trivedi SH, Burzynski JN, Schluger NW. Use of an interferon-γ release assay to

diagnose latent tuberculosis infection in foreign-born patients. Chest. 2008;**133**(4):869-874

[67] Kumar R, Das RK, Mahapatra AK. Role of interferon gamma release assay in the diagnosis of Pott disease. Journal of Neurosurgery. Spine. 2010;**12**(5):462-466

[68] Viswanathan VK, Subramanian S. Pott Disease. Treasure Island (FL): StatPearls Publishing; 2022. Available from: https://www.ncbi.nlm.nih.gov/books/NBK538331/

[69] Oguz E, Sehirlioglu A, Altinmakas M, Ozturk C, Komurcu M, Solakoglu C, et al. A new classification and guide for surgical treatment of spinal tuberculosis. International Orthopaedics. 2008;**32**(1):127-133

[70] Mehmet T, Ali A, Ahmet TT, Ravindra KG. Tuberculosis of the Central Nervous System. Aydin, Turkey: Springer US; 2017. pp. 195-219

[71] Wang Z, Shi J, Geng G, Qiu H. Ultra-short-course chemotherapy for spinal tuberculosis: Five years of observation. European Spine Journal. 2013;**22**(2):274-281

[72] Valsalan R, Purushothaman R, Raveendran MK, Zacharia B, Surendran S. Efficacy of directly observed treatment short-course intermittent regimen in spinal tuberculosis. Indian Journal of Orthopaedics. 2012;**46**(2):138-144

[73] Cox HS, Morrow M, Deutschmann PW. Long term efficacy of DOTS regimens for tuberculosis: Systematic review. BMJ. 2008;**336**(7642):484-487

[74] Jawahar MS. Current trends in chemotherapy of tuberculosis. The Indian Journal of Medical Research. 2004;**120**(4):398-417

[75] Bodapati P, Vemula RV, Mohammad A, Mohan A. Outcome and management of spinal tuberculosis according to severity at a tertiary referral center. Asian Journal of Neurosurgery. 2017;**12**(3):441

[76] Barclay WR, Ebert RH, Le Roy GV, Manthei RW, Roth LJ. Distribution and excretion of radioactive isoniazid in tuberculous patients. Journal of the American Medical Association. 1953;**151**(16):1384-1388. Available from: http://www.ncbi.nlm.nih.gov/pubmed/13034481

[77] Bosworth DM, Wright HA. Streptomycin in bone and joint tuberculosis. The Journal of Bone and Joint Surgery. American Volume. 1952; **34 A**(2):255-266

[78] Tuli SM. Judicious management of tuberculosis of bones joints and spine. Indian Journal of Orthopaedics. 2019;**19**(02):147. Available from: http://www.ijoonline.com/article.asp?issn=0019-5413;year=1985;volume=19;issue=02;spage=147;epage=166;aulast=Tuli;type=0

[79] Tuli SM. Results of treatment of spinal tuberculosis by "middle path" regime. Journal of Bone and Joint Surgery - Series B. 1975;**57**(1):13-23

[80] Tenth report of the Medical Research Council. A controlled trial of six-month and nine-month regimens of chemotherapy in patients undergoing radical surgery for tuberculosis of the spine in Hong Kong. Tubercle. 1986;**67**(4):243-259. Available from: http://www.ncbi.nlm.nih.gov/pubmed/2889281

[81] Tuli SM. Severe kyphotic deformity in tuberculosis of the spine. International Orthopaedics. 1995;**19**(5):327-331

[82] Hodgson AR, Stock FE. Anterior spinal fusion a preliminary

communication on the radical treatment of pott's disease and pott's paraplegia. The British Journal of Surgery. 1956;**44**(185):266-275

[83] Wimmer C. Perkutane dorsale Stabilisierung an der Brust- und Lendenwirbelsäule mit dem Expedium LIS. Operative Orthopädie und Traumatologie. 2008;**20**(6):511-524. Available from: http://www.ncbi.nlm.nih.gov/pubmed/19137398

[84] Abbas A, Rizvi SRH, Mahesri M, Salahuddin HRA. Conservative management of spinal tuberculosis: Initial series from Pakistan. Asian Spine Journal. 2013;7(2):73-80

[85] Benli IT, Kaya A, Acaroğlu E. Anterior instrumentation in tuberculous spondylitis: Is it effective and safe? Clinical Orthopaedics and Related Research. 2007;**460**:108-116

[86] Christodoulou AG, Givissis P, Karataglis D, Symeonidis PD, Pournaras J. Treatment of tuberculous spondylitis with anterior stabilization and titanium cage. Clinical Orthopaedics and Related Research. 2006;**444**:60-65

[87] Govender S, Kumar KPS. Cortical allografts in spinal tuberculosis. International Orthopaedics. 2003;**27**(4):244-248. DOI: 10.1007/s00264-003-0446-9. Available from: http://www.embase.com/search/results?subaction=viewrecord&from=export&id=L37070885%0A

[88] Moon MS. Tuberculosis of spine: Current views in diagnosis and management. Asian Spine Journal. 2014;**8**(1):97-111

[89] Jain AK, Dhammi IK, Prashad B, Sinha S, Mishra P. Simultaneous anterior decompression and posterior instrumentation of the tuberculous spine using an anterolateral extrapleural approach. Journal of Bone and Joint Surgery - Series B. 2008;**90**(11):1477-1481

[90] Zhong W, Xiong G, Wang B, Lu C, Dai Z, Lv G. Surgical management for thoracic spinal tuberculosis posterior only versus anterior video-assisted thoracoscopic surgery. PLoS One. 2015;**10**(3). DOI: 10.1371/journal.pone.0119759. Available from: http://www.embase.com/search/results?subaction=viewrecord&from=export&id=L603051675%0A

[91] Lee SH, Sung JK, Park YM. Single-stage transpedicular decompression and posterior instrumentation in treatment of thoracic and thoracolumbar spinal tuberculosis: A retrospective case series. Journal of Spinal Disorders & Techniques. 2006;**19**(8):595-602

[92] Chen YC, Chang MC, Wang ST, Yu WK, Liu CL, Chen TH. One-stage posterior surgery for treatment of advanced spinal tuberculosis. Journal of the Chinese Medical Association. 2003;**66**(7):411-417

[93] Chen WJ, Wu CC, Jung CH, Chen LH, Niu CC, Lai PL. Combined anterior and posterior surgeries in the treatment of spinal tuberculous spondylitis. Clinical Orthopaedics and Related Research. 2002;**398**(398):50-59. DOI: 10.1097/00003086-200205000-00008. Available from: http://www.embase.com/search/results?subaction=viewrecord&from=export&id=L34465324%0A

[94] Talu U, Gogus A, Ozturk C, Hamzaoglu A, Domanic U. The role of posterior instrumentation and fusion after anterior radical debridement and fusion in the surgical treatment of spinal tuberculosis: Experience of 127 cases. Journal of Spinal Disorders

& Techniques. 2006;**19**(8):554-559. DOI: 10.1097/01.bsd.0000211202.93125.c7. Available from: http://www.embase.com/search/results?subaction=viewrecord&from=export&id=L44912344%0A

[95] Colmenero JD, Ruiz-Mesa JD, Sanjuan-Jimenez R, Sobrino B, Morata P. Establishing the diagnosis of tuberculous vertebral osteomyelitis. European Spine Journal. 2013;**22**(Suppl. 4)

[96] Turgut M, Ozcan OE, Ozgen T, Saglam S, Bertan V, Erbengi A. Tuberculomas of the craniospinal axis. Turkish Neurosurgery. 1990;**1**(1):34-38

[97] Moore SL, Rafii M. Imaging of musculoskeletal and spinal tuberculosis. Radiologic Clinics of North America. 2001;**39**(2):329-342

[98] Zheng B, Hao D, Guo H, He B. Anterior versus posterior surgical approach for lumbosacral tuberculosis. The Journal of International Medical Research. 2018;**46**(7):2569-2577

[99] Rajasekaran S, Vijay K, Shetty AP. Single-stage closing-opening wedge osteotomy of spine to correct severe post-tubercular kyphotic deformities of the spine: A 3-year follow-up of 17 patients. European Spine Journal. 2010;**19**(4):583-592

[100] Kalra KP, Dhar SB, Shetty G, Dhariwal Q. Pedicle subtraction osteotomy for rigid post-tuberculous kyphosis. Journal of Bone and Joint Surgery - Series B. 2006;**88**(7):925-927

[101] Grevitt M, Kamath V, Avadhani A, Rajasekaran S. Correction of thoracic kyphosis with Ponte osteotomy. European Spine Journal. 2010;**19**(2):351-352

[102] Rajasekaran S. Natural history of Pott's kyphosis. European Spine Journal. 2013;**22**(Suppl.4):S634-S640. DOI: 10.1007/s00586-012-2336-6. Available from: http://www.embase.com/search/results?subaction=viewrecord&from=export&id=L52010388%0A

[103] Yusuf N, Ali MA, Ahmad Q, Rahman L, Nigar T. Pregnancy in Pott's disease: A case report and review. Bangladesh Journal of Obstetrics & Gynaecology. 2010;**25**(1):37-40

[104] Han IH, Kuh SU, Kim JH, Chin DK, Kim KS, Yoon YS, et al. Clinical approach and surgical strategy for spinal diseases in pregnant women: A report of ten cases. Spine (Phila Pa 1976). 2008;**33**(17):E614-E617. DOI: 10.1097/BRS.0b013e31817c6c7d. Available from: http://www.embase.com/search/results?subaction=viewrecord&from=export&id=L354648620%0A

[105] Kaul R, Chhabra HS, Kanagaraju V, Mahajan R, Tandon V, Nanda A, et al. Antepartum surgical management of Pott's paraplegia along with maintenance of pregnancy during second trimester. European Spine Journal. 2016;**25**(4):1064-1069

[106] Kaushal S, Dora SK, Thakur S. Spinal tuberculosis with paraplegia in pregnancy: A case report with management of spinal TB in pregnancy. Journal of Nepal Medical Association. 2015;**53**(198):123-125

[107] Hsu LCS, Leong JCY. Tuberculosis of the lower cervical spine (C2 to C7). A report on 40 cases. Journal of Bone and Joint Surgery - Series B. 1984;**66**(1):1-5

[108] Teo HE, Peh WC. Skeletal tuberculosis in children. Pediatric Radiology. 2004;**34**(11):853-860

[109] Behari S, Nayak SR, Bhargava V, Banerji D, Chhabra DK, Jain VK, et al. Craniocervical tuberculosis: Protocol

of surgical management. Neurosurgery. 2003;**52**(1):72-81

[110] Fisher T. Pulmonary tuberculosis in children. British Medical Journal. 1909;**1**(2512):504

[111] Upadhyay SS, Saji MJ, Yau ACMC. Duration of antituberculosis chemotherapy in conjunction with radical surgery in the management of spinal tuberculosis. Spine (Phila Pa 1976). 1996;**21**(16):1898-1903

[112] Rajeswari R, Balasubramanian R, Venkatesan P, Sivasubramanian S, Soundarapandian S, Shanmugasundaram TK, et al. Short-course chemotherapy in the treatment of Pott's paraplegia: Report on five year follow-up. The International Journal of Tuberculosis and Lung Disease. 1997;**1**(2):152-158

[113] Ruben F, Jacobs RF, O'Brien R, Bass JB, Hopewell PC, Farer LS, et al. Treatment of tuberculosis and tuberculosis infection in adults and children. American thoracic society and the centers for disease control and prevention. American Journal of Respiratory and Critical Care Medicine. 2013;**149**(5):1359-1374

[114] Benzagmout M, Boujraf S, Chakour K, Chaoui M. Potts disease in children. Surgical Neurology International. 2011;**2**(1)

[115] Ndiaye M, Sene-Diouf F, Diop AG, Sakho Y, Ndiaye MM, Ndiaye IP. Pott's spinal cord compression in the child. Dakar Médical. 1999;**44**(1):49-53

[116] Ha KY, Chung YG, Ryoo SJ. Adherence and biofilm formation of Staphylococcus Epidermidis and Mycobacterium Tuberculosis on various spinal implants. Spine (Phila Pa 1976). 2005;**30**(1):38-43

[117] Bin WX, Li J, Lü GH, Wang B, Lu C, Kang YJ. Single-stage posterior instrumentation and anterior debridement for active tuberculosis of the thoracic and lumbar spine with kyphotic deformity. International Orthopaedics. 2012;**36**(2):373-380

[118] Tuli SM, Kumar K, Sen PC. Penetration of antitubercular drugs in clinical osteoarticular tubercular lesions. Acta Orthopaedica. 1977;**48**(4):362-368

Chapter 5

Principles of Rehabilitation Strategies in Spinal Cord Injury

Seyed Mansoor Rayegani, Roozbeh Tavanaei and Saeed Oraee-Yazdani

Abstract

Spinal cord injury (SCI) is a debilitating condition that affects millions of people worldwide and results in a remarkable health economic burden imposed on patients and the healthcare system annually. The most common causes of SCI are the trauma caused by falls, traffic accidents, or violence. The course of SCI is associated with several complications that severely impair the patient's quality of life, including sensory and motor dysfunction, pain, neurogenic bladder and bowel, autonomic dysreflexia, cardiovascular and pulmonary dysfunction, spasticity, urinary tract infection, and sexual dysfunction. Despite great strides that have been made in the field of regenerative medicine and neural repair, the treatment of SCI still mostly revolves around rehabilitative strategies to improve patients' quality of life and function. Rehabilitation following the SCI is a multidisciplinary process that requires the involvement of multiple disciplines. Moreover, recent advances in the field of neurorehabilitation following SCI, are changing the face of this field. Therefore, we decided to review various aspects of rehabilitation following the SCI, including the goals and different modalities whereby we could achieve them.

Keywords: spinal cord injury, rehabilitation, paraplegia, restoration of function, quality of life

1. Introduction

Spinal cord injury (SCI) results from damage to the spinal cord, which could lead to significant temporary or permanent functional impairment. As a debilitating condition, SCI affects millions of people worldwide and imposes a considerable economic burden on patients and the healthcare system each year [1, 2]. Traumatic etiologies, such as traffic accidents, falls, and violence constitute the most common causes of SCI [2]. Throughout the course of SCI, various complications could severely impair the patients' quality of life (QoL) and activities of daily living (ADL) over the long term. These complications include sensory and motor dysfunction, pain, neurogenic bladder and bowel, autonomic dysreflexia, cardiovascular and pulmonary dysfunction, spasticity, urinary tract infection, and sexual dysfunction [3].

In recent decades, great strides have been made in the field of neuroregeneration to provide functional recovery through neural repair and axonal regrowth [4].

However, at present, there exists no definitive treatment modality to effectively restore spinal cord structural integrity following SCI with subsequent functional recovery. Therefore, the treatment of SCI still mostly revolves around rehabilitative strategies to improve patients' QoL and function [5, 6]. Rehabilitation following the SCI is a multidisciplinary process that requires the involvement of multiple disciplines, such as physiatrists, nurses, psychologists, dieticians, physical therapists, social workers, occupational therapists, orthotists and speech therapists [6, 7]. The rehabilitation process in SCI mostly centers around restoring the lost functions or augmenting the remaining intact functions while minimizing the associated complications. Holistic approach derived from biopsychosociospiritual model of health is essential for rehabilitation management of SCI. Functional restoration measures including mobility, strength, stretch and coordination training as well as cardiovascular and pulmonary rehabilitation constitute the main aspects of the rehabilitation process following SCI [6, 8].

In addition to current rehabilitation programs, recent advances in the field of neurorehabilitation for functional recovery, are changing the face of this field. Therefore, the focus of this chapter is on the goals of rehabilitation in SCI, current rehabilitative strategies, and recent advances in neurorehabilitation that have opened new horizons for patient management.

2. Goals of rehabilitation in spinal cord injury

The American Spinal Injury Association (ASIA) Impairment Scale (AIS) is a standardized tool for the classification of SCI patients based on injury severity and the level of sensorimotor impairment [9]. The AIS ranges from A (complete injury with no sensorimotor function preserved below the level of injury) to E (a normal sensorimotor function without neurological deficit). **Table 1** demonstrates details of AIS grading. Given its strong correlation with the functional status of the patient, AIS grade is one of the major factors in determining the functional goals of SCI patients following rehabilitation. In this regard, patients with complete SCI have a poorer prognosis for neurological recovery and improvement in functional outcomes compared to those with incomplete injury [10–13].

The neurological level of injury is another factor that affects the prognosis of SCI patients [14, 15]. In terms of motor recovery, patients with the cervical level of injury generally have a higher potential for functional improvement in comparison with those who have thoracic SCI. Moreover, among patients with cervical SCI, those who have an injury at lower cervical levels (C6-C8) show the greatest rehabilitation potential [6]. This is due mostly to remarkable functional impairment in upper cervical injuries and functional independence in many ADLs in thoracolumbar SCI patients, which reduces their potential for recovery. Concerning this, a number of patients with a high cervical level of injury (C3-C4) are ventilator-dependent and almost all of them are dependent to perform their ADLs. Patients with a C5 level of injury, although dependent on assistance for transferability, could perform ADLs, such as nutrition, dressing, and hygiene with assistance, given the preserved strength of elbow flexion in this group. Lower levels of cervical injury are generally associated with enough muscle strength for wrist extension, elbow extension, or finger flexion, which make patients in this group independent in most self-care ADLs and also transferring using assistive devices [6]. Patients with thoracic SCI, however, are totally independent in ADLs and transferability using a manual wheelchair. Thus, the main aim of rehabilitation in this group of patients

Grade A	No sensorimotor function
Grade B	Preserved sensory function with no motor function below the level of injury, which includes S4-S5 level
Grade C	Preserved motor function in more than half of the key muscles below the level of injury with a strength <3/5
Grade D	Preserved motor function in at least half of key muscles below the level of injury with a strength ≥3/5
Grade E	Normal sensorimotor function

Table 1.
The American spinal injury association (ASIA) impairment scale (AIS).

is ambulation. Patients with lower levels of injury (L1 or lower) show complete independence in ADLs and transferability in addition to an adequate degree of ambulation [6].

In addition to neurological recovery, early rehabilitation is necessary to prevent potential long-term complications [6]. As mentioned earlier, various complications affect the QoL in SCI patients, especially over the long term. Many interventions and strategies have been utilized in SCI rehabilitation to reduce the risk of chronic complications in patients with SCI. Recent advances in the field of SCI rehabilitation with the existing evidence have been discussed in the forthcoming paragraphs of this chapter based on different areas of rehabilitation.

3. Rehabilitation interventions

Multidisciplinary team approach is mainstay of SCI rehabilitation. In this model of rehabilitation an organized team including physician with expertise in rehabilitation that is usually a physical medicine and rehabilitation specialist (physiatris) as the team leader, physical therapist, occupational therapist, rehabilitation nurses, social worker, clinical psychologist, orthotists and dietician has the responsibility of planning, executing and follow up of rehabilitation measures. The team benefits from expertise skills of neurospine surgeon and other medical specialties as needed. Followings are more related and mostly used rehabilitation medicine measures that are used in management of SCI.

3.1 Sensorimotor dysfunction

3.1.1 Physical therapy

Physical therapy is one of the major measures of the post-SCI rehabilitation program and begins early in the course of SCI [6, 8, 16]. By targeting various aspects of impairment, such as strength, joint mobility, muscle extensibility, spasticity, pain, and cardiovascular fitness, physical therapy could improve patients' functional independence and prevent long-term complications. Range of motion and stretching exercises could prevent the development of contractures and protect the unwanted tenodesis effect [6]. Moreover, passive muscle stretching exercises could reduce muscle tone and help in maintaining the range of motion and joint mobility, which in turn decrease spasticity-related side effects.

3.1.2 Orthoses and assistive devices

Orthoses could also be used to position the joints and prevent contracture formation [6, 17, 18]. Strengthening exercises for intact regions are of great importance, particularly in patients with complete paraplegia during the early period of rehabilitation, to provide adequate strength for independent mobilization and transferability. Assistive devices, such as a wheelchair, walker, or crutch might also be utilized depending on the functional status of patients for ambulation during the chronic rehabilitation period [6].

3.1.3 Transcranial direct current stimulation

Transcranial direct current stimulation (tDCS) is a noninvasive modality that is used to modify cortical excitability by delivering weak electrical currents (1–2 mA). The tDCS consists of anodal and cathodal electrodes, which following their application, could increase and suppress cortical excitability [19, 20]. The main concept behind the use of tDCS in SCI is modulation of the excitability of residual cortical motor pathways to enhance functional recovery. Previous individual studies have demonstrated promising potential for tDCS combined with various rehabilitative strategies in improving motor cortex excitability and muscle power [21–24]. However, a meta-analysis including six studies and 78 patients with SCI found no significant efficacy for tDCS in increasing muscle strength in comparison with sham tDCS [25]. Moreover, based on their findings, the effect of tDCS on motor functional improvement was marginally significant with a small effect size. In addition, their subgroup analyses failed to demonstrate any significant association between cortical area (hand or leg motor cortex), additional interventions (tDCS alone or tDCS combined with other interventions), or tDCS intensity (1 or 2 mA) the impact of tDCS on outcomes observed in patients. Nevertheless, the limited number of studies, as well as the heterogeneity in methods and protocols among existing investigations have mostly resulted in inconclusive results regarding the efficacy of tDCS in SCI. Therefore, future high-quality studies are highly demanded to show the potential effectiveness of tDCS in improving motor outcomes in SCI patients. Further, some of characteristics, such as non-invasiveness and cost-effectiveness, make tDCS a great potential therapeutic option for SCI.

3.1.4 Repetitive transcranial magnetic stimulation

Transcranial magnetic stimulation (TMS) is another safe and non-invasive cortical stimulation method for modulating neuronal excitability. In this technique, following the passage of the electrical current through a coil, which is placed on the scalp, short magnetic fields are generated. These magnetic fields subsequently induce electrical pulses in neurons, which act as secondary coils [26]. One single TMS pulse over the primary motor cortex elicits action potentials in a group of neurons, which induce motor evoked potential (MEP) in the corresponding muscle group, depending on the topographic area stimulated [26]. Considering this effect, the delivery of several pulses using TMS in a sequential order could exert long-term changes in neuroplasticity-related mechanisms, such as long-term potentiation or depression [27, 28]. This specific TMS modality is known as repetitive TMS (rTMS). Based on stimulation parameters, rTMS could either increase (facilitatory) or decrease (inhibitory) cortical excitability [26]. The therapeutic efficacy of rTMS is well-established in some psychological disorders, such as depression. Moreover, a huge body of evidence has demonstrated significant effects of rTMS on motor recovery following stroke [29]. With respect to SCI, however, limited evidence exists especially on the effects of rTMS on sensorimotor recovery [30]. Previous investigations have demonstrated significant improvements in lower extremities motor scores following the use of high-frequency rTMS compared with the sham stimulation in patients with SCI [31–35]. One study also demonstrated an average increase of 40–50% in the amplitude of corticospinal responses and magnitude of maximal voluntary contractions in targeted muscles after paired stimulation using both rTMS and peripheral nerve stimulation in patients with SCI [36]. In addition to sensorimotor recovery, the effects of rTMS on SCI-induced spasticity and neuropathic pain have also been evaluated. Two recent meta-analyses and systematic reviews, one including 10 randomized controlled trials (RCTs) and one evaluating 6 RCTs, demonstrated a significant reduction in SCI-induced neuropathic pain intensity in patients who received rTMS compared with the control group [37, 38]. Some prior studies have also reported significant improvements in spasticity following the SCI in patients receiving rTMS [31, 33, 34]. However, as mentioned earlier, given the existing heterogeneity among these studies regarding the rTMS parameters, further evidence is highly demanded.

3.1.5 Deep brain stimulation

Deep brain stimulation (DBS) is a minimally invasive neurosurgical procedure, which includes adjustable stimulation of specific target parts of the brain through implanted electrodes, and is widely implemented for the treatment of movement disorders [39]. Recently, however, DBS has received attention as a potential option for motor functional recovery in SCI. The electrical activation of preserved sublesional descending motor pathways such as the reticulospinal tract forms the rationale behind the potential use of DBS in SCI. In this regard, previous preclinical investigations have demonstrated significant improvement in deficient gait due to SCI and stroke following the stimulation of the mesencephalic locomotor region (MLR) in animal models [40–42]. In a previous study, acute excitatory DBS of the MLR resulted in remarkably improved motor function of the paretic hindlimb in a rat model of chronic incomplete SCI [40]. Moreover, significant improvements in dynamic gait parameters and walking speed have also been reported with high-frequency DBS of the MLR in the rat stroke model [41]. An ongoing clinical trial (NCT03053791) is currently recruiting patients to evaluate the potential effects of MLR-DBS in SCI patients for the first time [43]. This therapeutic modality with its application in SCI is still at its initial stages, and further research is required to elucidate various aspects of it, especially underlying mechanisms, and translate it to the clinical setting.

3.1.6 Epidural spinal cord stimulation

One form of spinal cord stimulation (SCS) is epidural SCS (eSCS), which includes surgical implantation of an array of electrodes over the dorsal surface of the spinal cord in the epidural space with direct stimulation of dorsal nerve roots. Initially, eSCS was evaluated for its impact on chronic pain due to its neuromodulatory effects on nociceptive afferent. Subsequent investigations showed that eSCS could also improve motor functional independence in chronic SCI patients through stimulating dorsal nerve roots and activating interneuronal pathways associated with locomotion [44]. Initial reports demonstrated that eSCS could restore independent standing with volitional control of lower limb activity and independent stepping in patients with complete SCI [45–47]. In another report including four patients, following multiple sessions of eSCS with gait training, all patients achieved independent standing and trunk stability, and two could walk on the ground [48]. Wagner et al. showed that spatiotemporal stimulation of the lumbosacral spinal cord using an implanted pulse generator in patients with chronic SCI could restore adaptive control of muscles and improve locomotion following rehabilitation [49]. In a recent study, the same research group demonstrated the restoration of a number of activities, including standing, walking, cycling, swimming, and trunk control, in three patients with complete sensorimotor paralysis using eSCS, as part of a clinical trial (NCT02936453) [50]. In this study, the optimal position of the paddle lead was determined using a computational framework to allow for the restoration of various motor activities using different activity-specific programs. In addition, there is preclinical evidence regarding the improvements in upper limb function, such as reaching and grasping following the use of cervical eSCS in cervical SCI [51]. A prior study, including two patients with chronic cervical SCI, also demonstrated improved hand strength and volitional hand control using cervical eSCS [52].

3.1.7 Transcutaneous spinal cord stimulation

Similar to eSCS, transcutaneous spinal cord stimulation (tcSCS) activates spinal motor pathways through stimulating dorsal root afferents, yet in a non-invasive manner [53]. In tcSCS, electrodes are generally placed on the skin overlying lower thoracic or lumbar vertebrae. The increase in excitability of local interneuronal pathways following the use of tcSCS facilitates the activity of previously spared nonfunctional supraspinal pathways [54]. This could lead to significant functional improvement, particularly in combination with other conventional rehabilitation strategies. Some previous reports have indicated improved postural control and ankle motility in patients with complete or incomplete SCI [55, 56]. A previous study showed improvements in weight loading capacity and reduced gait asymmetry in 19 patients who received exoskeleton-based training with tcSCS [57]. There are other studies reporting significantly enhanced volitional lower extremity movement, walking speed, endurance, and symmetry using tcSCS combined with walking and locomotion training [58–60]. In regard to the upper limb, similarly, a number of studies have demonstrated significant durable improvements in upper extremity function, such as grip force and dexterity following tcSCS with training [61, 62]. Based on prior findings, tcSCS results in a functional recovery sustained over periods without stimulation. Therefore, given the speed of acquisition, it has been proposed that tcSCS might be associated with a broader modulatory effect on neuronal pathways compared with eSCS, which merely causes a transient increase in excitability [53]. Despite being non-invasive and inexpensive, tcSCS has a remarkably lower spatiotemporal precision than eSCS. Current literature on the utility of tcSCS in SCI is heterogeneous, especially in terms of stimulation parameters, study design, and outcome measures. Hence, future high-quality clinical trials with larger sample sizes are highly needed in this regard.

3.1.8 Functional electrical stimulation

Functional electrical stimulation (FES) is a widely used neurorehabilitation modality in which electrical stimulation of the paralyzed muscles is performed to achieve functional improvement. During FES sessions, generally, neuromuscular stimulation is contemporaneous with specific tasks, such as cycling [63]. Previous studies have demonstrated that FES is associated with improved circulation, muscle strength, range of motion, and reduced spasticity [64]. Various activities have been evaluated in previous studies on FES, including cycling, walking, grasping, reaching, and stair climbing [63]. FES-evoked cycling is one of the most frequently used FES training modalities in the clinical setting [64, 65]. In this rehabilitation method, patients with no or reduced volitional lower extremity control can perform cycling using an exercise bicycle. The pedaling motion is produced by computer-generated electrical pulses that are transmitted to leg muscles through surface electrodes. Several benefits have been previously reported for FES cycling, including significant improvements in motor scores, functional independence, spasticity, and cardiopulmonary function in SCI patients [63, 64, 66, 67]. A recent systematic review evaluated 99 studies, including 999 SCI patients, and suggested that FES cycling exercise could improve lower-body muscle health, power output, and aerobic fitness in SCI patients [64]. With respect to the upper limb, prior studies have also reported better recovery in hand function in cervical SCI patients receiving FES, especially when combined with conventional occupational therapy [68, 69]. Electrical pulses in FES are defined mainly based on three parameters, including pulse frequency (typical values, 20–50 Hz), amplitude (typical values, 0–100 mA), and width (typical values, 300–600 μs) [63]. Differences in parameter adjustments significantly change the effects of FES on muscle contraction and fatigue. Therefore, depending on the rehabilitation goals and the patient's functional status, parameters could be individualized.

3.1.9 Transcutaneous electrical nerve stimulation

Transcutaneous electrical nerve stimulation (TENS) is a non-invasive and safe rehabilitation modality whereby electrical pulses are delivered to the skin to stimulate nerves and reduce pain subsequently. Based on prior findings, a remarkable increase in blood circulation following TENS results in pain improvement [70–73]. Various clinical conditions could be targeted through differences in electrode placement and stimulation parameters, including frequency and intensity [73, 74]. The frequency of stimulation could be high (>50 Hz) or low (<10 Hz). The stimulation intensity is also classified based on the response achieved, which could be sensory or motor. The use of TENS in pain treatment is well-studied and mostly consists of delivering low-frequency electrical pulses to the affected area. A recent meta-analysis, including six RCTs with 165 patients, indicated that visual analog scale (VAS) for pain and short-form McGill pain questionnaire scores were significantly reduced in SCI patients who received TENS compared with the control group [75]. In addition to pain, prior evidence supports the use of TENS in improving spasticity [76]. Regarding this, a previous systematic review and meta-analysis demonstrated a significant association between the TENS applied for more than 30 minutes and reduction in lower limb spasticity in patients with chronic stroke [77]. Similarly, a number of previous studies have reported significant improvements in SCI-induced spasticity using TENS [78–80]. Given its safety profile and low cost as well as effects on pain and spasticity, TENS is regarded as a great adjunct to physical therapy and conventional SCI rehabilitation program.

3.1.10 Robotic-assisted gait training

In addition to reduced functional independence, immobility due to SCI could lead to a variety of secondary problems, including cardiopulmonary complications, bowel and bladder dysfunction, osteoporosis, pressure ulcers, and obesity [81–83]. Accordingly, recovery of ambulation is of crucial importance in the rehabilitation program of patients with SCI [84]. Locomotor rehabilitation training following the SCI is performed either in a conventional manner, in which the therapist assists manually, or by using rehabilitation robots, which are also known as exoskeletons. In comparison with the former, robotic-assisted gait training is associated with a less physical burden for the therapist while also allowing for quantitative evaluation of the patient's progression [85–92]. Since the introduction of Lokomat, as the first exoskeleton, different types of gait rehabilitation robots have been developed [92, 93]. Many prior studies have evaluated the effects of robotic-assisted gait training in SCI rehabilitation. Several beneficial impacts for this modality have been reported previously, including improvements in musculoskeletal, urinary, cardiopulmonary, somatosensory, and neural plasticity [87, 89, 94, 95]. Based on a previous systematic review, including 13 RCTs, body weight-supported treadmill training and robotic-assisted gait training increase the walking speed no more than overground gait training and other forms of physical therapy in patients with SCI [90]. However, the results were not clear regarding the changes in walking distance. Another systematic review and meta-analysis, including 10 RCTs, found that robotic-assisted gait training results in significantly greater improvement in mobility-related outcomes, such as gait distance, functional level of mobility and independence, and leg strength compared with conventional overground training in incomplete SCI patients [87]. Nevertheless, potential differences in response to therapy between different individuals with SCI should also be considered. Concerning this, patients with incomplete lesions or a recent injury might show a better response to therapy with robotic-assisted gait training than those with complete or chronic injuries [90]. Thus, future trials are warranted to allow for further subgroups analyses in this regard. Furthermore, recently, wearable exoskeletons, as emerging therapeutic devices are receiving much attention since they require active participation from the patient and could also be utilized as assistive devices in the community [92]. Additionally, wearable exoskeletons seem to address limitations associated with grounded exoskeletons by providing more freedom during gait and the ability to perform complex motions and more activities of daily living. However, since there is a paucity of data regarding various aspects of wearable exoskeletons and their effectiveness in patients with SCI, future clinical trials are highly warranted to evaluate the utility of different robots and also compare them with other types of gait therapy in this population [92].

3.1.11 Occupational therapy

One of the important disciplines in rehabilitation team of SCI is occupational therapy.

A person's functional independence has a major impact on their quality of life, and consequential social participation. Some people with a spinal cord injury (SCI) will have the ability to achieve a high level of independence while others, limited by their physical ability, will be able to achieve a level of independence through directing their care and by using technology options. Whilst it is reasonable to expect that the degree of functional independence achievable is dependent on a person's level of injury, a person's neurological level should not be viewed as strictly predictive but rather as indicative of potential function. Adjustment of SCI with post injury functional limitation and activity of daily living (ADL) copping is very essential for victims of SCI. Transfer activities, transportation from and to different environments, home adjustments and copping to new adjusted work are among professional activities of occupational therapist in rehabilitation team. In addition, neurorehabilitation facilitations techniques such as anti-spasticity manures are carried out by occupational therapists.

3.2 Cardiopulmonary dysfunction

Recent advances in the care and rehabilitation of SCI patients have changed the pattern of SCI morbidity and mortality with a shift from septicemia, pneumonia, and renal failure to cardiovascular complications as one of the major causes of death in this group of patients [96, 97]. Many risk factors for cardiovascular disease are associated with SCI, including physical inactivity due to the non-ambulatory state, extreme fluctuations in blood pressure, dyslipidemia, abnormal glycemic control, and chronic inflammation [98, 99]. With respect to this, a previous survey with a large sample of 60,000 SCI patients showed a significant association between SCI and increased odds of heart disease and stroke [96].

In addition, numerous previous investigations have reported a high prevalence of orthostatic hypotension in SCI [100, 101]. Similar to acute injury, orthostatic hypotension could be persistent throughout the course of chronic SCI and remarkably interfere with the rehabilitation process and patient's QoL [100]. Improvements in orthostatic hypotension have been reported previously through a variety of measures, including pressure interventions (e.g., pressure stockings and abdominal binders), increasing fluid and salt intake (volume augmentation), lower limb FES, exercise, and pharmacotherapy using different agents, such as midodrine, fludrocortisone, ephedrine, dihydroergotamine, and droxidopa [100].

Autonomic dysreflexia is also an urgent cardiovascular condition associated with SCI, which is characterized by acute episodes of hypertension with either bradycardia or tachycardia [102, 103]. Most patients with a T6 level of injury or higher are at risk of autonomic dysreflexia. Various noxious and non-noxious stimuli below the level of injury, such as pressure sores, and bladder or bowel irritation, could lead to autonomic dysreflexia mainly by triggering massive sympathetic discharge. The clinical manifestation of autonomic dysreflexia is variable and ranges from mild discomfort to severe acute hypertension with ominous consequences [102, 103]. Prior reports have shown a significant correlation between the severity of autonomic dysreflexia and the level of injury, as well as the completeness of the SCI with higher and complete injuries are associated with more severe manifestations [102, 104]. Prevention plays a crucial role in the management of autonomic dysreflexia and mainly aims at resolving the underlying triggers through several non-pharmacologic measures, such as regular bladder and bowel care. Depending on the severity, pharmacologic therapy with rapid-onset antihypertensive drugs is also used in acute cases of autonomic dysreflexia [102].

Pulmonary dysfunction also noticeably complicates the course of SCI, particularly in patients with cervical and upper thoracic injuries. Functional impairments in respiratory muscles, including the diaphragm, intercostal, and accessory respiratory muscles, substantially reduce lung capacity and increase respiratory demand. Moreover, atelectasis ensues when the dysfunction of respiratory muscles leads to reduced compliance of the lung and chest wall. Impaired function of expiratory muscles also causes ineffective cough, which in turn negatively affects airway clearance. Consequently, many severe complications could occur as a result of pulmonary dysfunction, such as mucus retention, pleural effusion, pneumonia, and respiratory failure [105, 106]. Therefore, pulmonary rehabilitation is a vital part of the SCI rehabilitation program to prevent respiratory complications in patients [106]. Prior investigations have shown that respiratory muscle training effectively improves respiratory muscle strength and subsequently reduces respiratory complications in SCI patients [107–113]. Among subgroups of SCI patients, greater improvement in respiratory function following the rehabilitation has been reported in patients with tetraplegia and subacute injury [109]. Respiratory muscle training involves increasing the load on respiratory muscles, and different types of it have been reported previously, such as the use of resistive and threshold trainers, singing training, and normocapnic hyperpnoea [107].

3.3 Bladder and bowel dysfunction

Bladder and bowel dysfunction involves a significant proportion of patients following SCI and remarkably impairs their QoL. Genitourinary infections constitute the most common cause of re-hospitalization in SCI patients with about 30% of them being hospitalized annually. Moreover, the fifth most common cause of mortality in SCI patients, is genitourinary infection. Bowel dysfunction is the fourth leading cause of re-hospitalization and the second most common complication according to SCI patients [114–116]. Therefore, bladder and bowel care comprise a notable part of the SCI rehabilitation program.

Based on a prior report, about 77% of SCI patients lack the ability to void voluntarily, which makes them dependent on assistance [117]. The most common bladder drainage method for neurogenic bladder management with the lowest risk of complications and urinary tract infection in SCI patients is clean intermittent catheterization [114, 118]. Tetraplegic patients, however, might use indwelling or suprapubic catheters, which could increase the risk of complications, such as infection. Other techniques, such as Credé and Valsalva maneuvers might also be helpful in addition to primary drainage methods. Pharmacological therapy using anticholinergics or beta-3-agonists is also effective in reducing the intravesical pressure in cases with hyperreflexic detrusor. In refractory cases or patients with renal impairment, a number of procedures, such as intravesical botulinum-A toxin injection, surgical interventions (e.g., bladder reconstruction and diversion procedures), and sacral neuromodulation, might also help in improving the symptoms [114].

According to SCI patients, about 95% of them have chronic constipation, and 75% have experienced fecal incontinence, which could significantly affect various aspects of QoL and the social life of patients. Further, several complications might occur as a result of chronic constipation, including anal fissures, rectal bleeding, hemorrhoids, autonomic dysreflexia, and urinary tract infection [114, 119]. Therefore, SCI rehabilitation should include an individualized bowel management program aimed at regular bowel emptying, maintaining functional continence, and preventing potential complications [114, 119]. Conservative management in neurogenic bowel includes diet, abdominal massage, drinking a warm liquid before bowel care, digital rectal stimulation, and using stimulant suppositories. Further, there might be an additional need for pharmacological therapy using oral or rectal laxatives, especially in older patients or those with longstanding SCI [114, 120, 121]. For maintenance of stool consistency, bulking agents and stool softeners might also be used regularly. In addition, prucalopride is a prokinetic agent, which is used for chronic constipation due to neurogenic bowel [114]. In case of inadequate response to conservative therapy, invasive procedures, such as intestinal diversion (e.g., ileostomy or colostomy), Malone anterograde continence enema could significantly improve the patients' QoL [114, 122].

3.4 Neuropathic pain

Pain is one of the most common disabling complications following the SCI, which could significantly impair the patient's QoL [123–125]. According to prior information, the prevalence of pain among patients with SCI is about 65 to 85%, and approximately one-third of them report severe pain [126]. Based on International Spinal Cord Injury Pain (ISCIP) classification and underlying mechanisms, SCI-related pain is classically divided into nociceptive and neuropathic categories [127]. Nociceptive pain originates from nociceptors with preserved sensory innervation and could be either musculoskeletal or visceral. Analgesics, such as nonsteroidal anti-inflammatory drugs (NSAIDs) or opioids, could significantly improve nociceptive pain [127]. Neuropathic pain, however, is the most common type of pain in SCI patients with no definitive therapy due to its more complex etiology, which is still not well understood [128]. Neuropathic pain mainly arises from the disease of the somatosensory system and could occur either at the level of injury or below it. Relative to the neurological level of injury, the former type is defined as the pain within the distribution of one rostral and three caudal dermatomes. The below-level pain, however, is localized below the three dermatomes caudal to the neurological level of injury. Neuropathic pain might also be associated with sensory phenomena in the painful area, such as allodynia, which is defined as pain triggered by non-noxious stimuli (e.g., light touch), especially in the at-level pain category [127]. Given the complexity of neuropathic pain, many pharmacological and non-pharmacological therapeutic interventions have been utilized previously with variable efficacy and safety profiles. Pharmacological therapy using antiepileptics, tricyclic antidepressants, opioids, and cannabinoids has been reported. In refractory cases, non-pharmacological interventions, such as intrathecal drug administration, nerve blocks, dorsal root entry zone (DREZ) ablation procedures, SCS, tDCS, transcranial electrical stimulation (TES), and TMS might be beneficial [129].

3.5 Spasticity

Spasticity is one of the most common complications following injuries to upper motor neurons, such as SCI. Approximately 65% of SCI patients show symptoms of spasticity following their discharge from the acute rehabilitation program, and about 93% of those in the community are affected [130, 131]. As a sensorimotor control disorder due to upper motor neuron lesion, spasticity is presented as a velocity-dependent increase in tonic stretch reflex with clonus, spasms, and hyperreflexia [18]. About 35% of chronic SCI patients have problematic spasticity, which is defined as spasticity leading to functional limitation or requires antispasticity treatment [131, 132]. SCI-related spasticity shows a gradual course, which begins following the areflexia associated with the spinal shock period. Incomplete SCI and preserved sensorimotor function below the level of injury are associated with severe spasticity. SCI-related spasticity could significantly affect the patient's QoL and limit ADLs. Moreover, poorly treated spasticity results in pain, contractures, and skin breakdown, which interferes with the rehabilitation process and could also prevent neurological recovery [18, 130, 131]. Due mainly to the more diffuse pattern of SCI-induced spasticity in comparison with other pathologies, such as stroke or traumatic brain injury, regional or systemic therapies are preferred in SCI [18, 130]. Initial therapy for SCI-induced spasticity consists of physical therapy and pharmacological treatment. However, often the approaches fail to manage spasticity in SCI patients, or intolerable side effects due to pharmacological therapy occur, and further treatment modalities might be required. Intrathecal administration of baclofen using an implantable pump has been significantly effective in reducing intractable SCI-induced spasticity. However, this method is associated with some limitations, such as surgical complications, pump failure, and infections [133, 134]. Depending on the status of the patient, other modalities might also be used, such as local chemodenervation using phenol, ethanol, or botulinum toxin. Surgical interventions, such as selective dorsal rhizotomy, tenotomy, tendon lengthening and transfers might also be used in selected severe cases [18, 130].

4. Conclusions

This chapter reviewed different modalities and strategies used in the field of neurorehabilitation for SCI and various aspects of it, specifically. The process of rehabilitation is time-consuming and requires the participation of multiple disciplines as well as the patients and their family. In addition, in many cases, the use of each modality individually might not result in a discernible improvement. Therefore, it is of paramount importance to consider a combinatorial approach to SCI rehabilitation with the aim of improvement in patients' function and QoL using all the available options. Moreover, a notable number of strategies for neurological recovery in SCI were not covered, mainly because they were beyond the scope of this chapter. Recent advances in different fields, such as brain-machine interface, stem cell therapy, tissue engineering, gene therapy, exosomes, and optogenetics, have shown promising results in various aspects of SCI, both preclinically and clinically. However, still, further research is needed to translate these potentially effective modalities into the clinical arena and use them as part of the rehabilitation plan.

Author details

Seyed Mansoor Rayegani[1], Roozbeh Tavanaei[2] and Saeed Oraee-Yazdani[2*]

1 Physical Medicine and Rehabilitation Research Center, Shahid Beheshti University of Medical Sciences, Tehran, Iran

2 Functional Neurosurgery Research Center, Shohada Tajrish Comprehensive Neurosurgical Center of Excellence, Shahid Beheshti University of Medical Sciences, Tehran, Iran

*Address all correspondence to: saeed_o_yazdani@sbmu.ac.ir

References

[1] McDaid D, Park A-L, Gall A, et al. Understanding and modelling the economic impact of spinal cord injuries in the United Kingdom. Spinal Cord. 2019;**57**:778-788

[2] Singh A, Tetreault L, Kalsi-Ryan S, et al. Global prevalence and incidence of traumatic spinal cord injury. Clinical Epidemiology. 2014;**6**:309

[3] Simpson LA, Eng JJ, Hsieh JTC, et al. The health and life priorities of individuals with spinal cord injury: A systematic review. Journal of Neurotrauma. 2012;**29**:1548-1555

[4] Ashammakhi N, Kim H-J, Ehsanipour A, et al. Regenerative therapies for spinal cord injury. Tissue Engineering. Part B, Reviews. 2019;**25**:471-491

[5] Pizzolato C, Gunduz MA, Palipana D, et al. Non-invasive approaches to functional recovery after spinal cord injury: Therapeutic targets and multimodal device interventions. Experimental Neurology. 2021;**339**:113612

[6] Nas K, Yazmalar L, Şah V, et al. Rehabilitation of spinal cord injuries. World Journal of Orthopedics. 2015;**6**:8

[7] Ahuja CS, Wilson JR, Nori S, et al. Traumatic spinal cord injury. Nature Reviews Disease Primers. 2017;**3**:17018

[8] Gómara-Toldrà N, Sliwinski M, Dijkers MP. Physical therapy after spinal cord injury: A systematic review of treatments focused on participation. The Journal of Spinal Cord Medicine. 2014;**37**:371-379

[9] Kirshblum SC, Waring W, Biering-Sorensen F, et al. Reference for the 2011 revision of the international standards for neurological classification of spinal cord injury. The Journal of Spinal Cord Medicine. 2011;**34**:547-554

[10] Scivoletto G, Tamburella F, Laurenza L, et al. Who is going to walk? A review of the factors influencing walking recovery after spinal cord injury. Frontiers in Human Neuroscience. 2014;**8**:141

[11] Kay ED, Deutsch A, Wuermser LA. Predicting walking at discharge from inpatient rehabilitation after a traumatic spinal cord injury. Archives of Physical Medicine and Rehabilitation. 2007;**88**:745-750

[12] van Middendorp JJ, Hosman AJF, Donders ART, et al. A clinical prediction rule for ambulation outcomes after traumatic spinal cord injury: A longitudinal cohort study. Lancet. 2011;**377**:1004-1010

[13] Kirshblum S, Millis S, McKinley W, et al. Late neurologic recovery after traumatic spinal cord injury. Archives of Physical Medicine and Rehabilitation. 2004;**85**:1811-1817

[14] Waters RL, Yakura JS, Adkins RH, et al. Recovery following complete paraplegia. Archives of Physical Medicine and Rehabilitation. 1992;**73**:784-789

[15] Coleman WP, Geisler FH. Injury severity as primary predictor of outcome in acute spinal cord injury: Retrospective results from a large multicenter clinical trial. The Spine Journal. 2004;**4**:373-378

[16] Fu J, Wang H, Deng L, et al. Exercise training promotes functional recovery after spinal cord injury. Neural Plasticity. 2016;**2016**:4039580

[17] Diong J, Harvey LA, Kwah LK, et al. Incidence and predictors of contracture after spinal cord injury--a prospective cohort study. Spinal Cord. 2012;**50**:579-584

[18] Elbasiouny SM, Moroz D, Bakr MM, et al. Management of Spasticity after Spinal Cord Injury: Current techniques and future directions. Neurorehabilitation and Neural Repair. 2010;**24**:23

[19] Nitsche MA, Seeber A, Frommann K, et al. Modulating parameters of excitability during and after transcranial direct current stimulation of the human motor cortex. The Journal of Physiology. 2005;**568**:291-303

[20] Nitsche MA, Cohen LG, Wassermann EM, et al. Transcranial direct current stimulation: State of the art 2008. Brain Stimulation. 2008;**1**:206-223

[21] Gomes-Osman J, Field-Fote EC. Cortical vs. afferent stimulation as an adjunct to functional task practice training: A randomized, comparative pilot study in people with cervical spinal cord injury. Clinical Rehabilitation. 2014;**29**:771-782

[22] Potter-Baker KA, Janini DP, Lin Y-L, et al. Transcranial direct current stimulation (tDCS) paired with massed practice training to promote adaptive plasticity and motor recovery in chronic incomplete tetraplegia: A pilot study. The Journal of Spinal Cord Medicine. 2018;**41**:503-517

[23] Yozbatiran N, Keser Z, Davis M, et al. Transcranial direct current stimulation (tDCS) of the primary motor cortex and robot-assisted arm training in chronic incomplete cervical spinal cord injury: A proof of concept sham-randomized clinical study. NeuroRehabilitation. 2016;**39**:401-411

[24] Cortes M, Medeiros AH, Gandhi A, et al. Improved grasp function with transcranial direct current stimulation in chronic spinal cord injury. NeuroRehabilitation. 2017;**41**:51-59

[25] de Araújo AVL, Ribeiro FPG, Massetti T, et al. Effectiveness of anodal transcranial direct current stimulation to improve muscle strength and motor functionality after incomplete spinal cord injury: A systematic review and meta-analysis. Spinal Cord. 2020;**58**:635-646

[26] Hallett M. Transcranial magnetic stimulation: a primer. Neuron. 2007;**55**:187-199

[27] Suppa A, Huang Y-Z, Funke K, et al. Ten years of theta burst stimulation in humans: Established knowledge, Unknowns and Prospects. Brain Stimulation. 2016;**9**:323-335

[28] Chervyakov AV, Chernyavsky AY, Sinitsyn DO, et al. Possible mechanisms underlying the therapeutic effects of transcranial magnetic stimulation. Frontiers in Human Neuroscience. 2015;**9**:303

[29] Xiang H, Sun J, Tang X, et al. The effect and optimal parameters of repetitive transcranial magnetic stimulation on motor recovery in stroke patients: A systematic review and meta-analysis of randomized controlled trials. Clinical Rehabilitation. 2019;**33**:847-864

[30] Tazoe T, Perez MA. Effects of repetitive transcranial magnetic stimulation on recovery of function after spinal cord injury. Archives of Physical Medicine and Rehabilitation. 2015;**96**:S145-S155

[31] Benito J, Kumru H, Murillo N, et al. Motor and gait improvement in patients with incomplete spinal cord injury induced by high-frequency repetitive transcranial magnetic stimulation. Top Spinal Cord Injury Rehabilitation. 2012;**18**:106-112

[32] Krogh S, Aagaard P, Jønsson AB, et al. Effects of repetitive transcranial magnetic stimulation on recovery in lower limb muscle strength and gait function following spinal cord injury: A randomized controlled trial. Spinal Cord. 2022;**60**:135-141

[33] Kumru H, Murillo N, Samso JV, et al. Reduction of spasticity with repetitive transcranial magnetic stimulation in patients with spinal cord injury. Neurorehabilitation and Neural Repair. 2010;**24**:435-441

[34] Nardone R, Höller Y, Thomschewski A, et al. rTMS modulates reciprocal inhibition in patients with traumatic spinal cord injury. Spinal Cord. 2014;**52**:831-835

[35] Kumru H, Benito-Penalva J, Valls-Sole J, et al. Placebo-controlled study of rTMS combined with Lokomat(®) gait training for treatment in subjects with motor incomplete spinal cord injury. Experimental Brain Research. 2016;**234**:3447-3455

[36] Jo HJ, Perez MA. Corticospinal-motor neuronal plasticity promotes exercise-mediated recovery in humans with spinal cord injury. Brain. 2020;**143**:1368-1382

[37] Saleh C, Ilia TS, Jaszczuk P, et al. Is transcranial magnetic stimulation as treatment for neuropathic pain in patients with spinal cord injury efficient? A systematic review. Neurological Science Official Journal of Italian Neurology Society Italy Society Clinical Neurophysiology. 2022;**43**:3007-3018

[38] Li L, Huang H, Yu Y, et al. Non-invasive brain stimulation for neuropathic pain after spinal cord injury: A systematic review and network meta-analysis. Frontiers in Neuroscience. 2021;**15**:800560

[39] Hartmann CJ, Fliegen S, Groiss SJ, et al. An update on best practice of deep brain stimulation in Parkinson's disease. Therapeutic Advances in Neurological Disorders. 2019;**12**:1756286419838096

[40] Bachmann LC, Matis A, Lindau NT, et al. Deep brain stimulation of the midbrain locomotor region improves paretic hindlimb function after spinal cord injury in rats. Science Translational Medicine. 2013;**5**:208ra146

[41] Fluri F, Malzahn U, Homola GA, et al. Stimulation of the mesencephalic locomotor region for gait recovery after stroke. Annals of Neurology. 2017;**82**:828-840

[42] Bonizzato M, James ND, Pidpruzhnykova G, et al. Multi-pronged neuromodulation intervention engages the residual motor circuitry to facilitate walking in a rat model of spinal cord injury. Nature Communications. 2021;**12**:1925

[43] Stieglitz LH, Hofer A-S, Bolliger M, et al. Deep brain stimulation for locomotion in incomplete human spinal cord injury (DBS-SCI): Protocol of a prospective one-armed multi-Centre study. BMJ Open. 2021;**11**:e047670

[44] Eisdorfer JT, Smit RD, Keefe KM, et al. Epidural electrical stimulation: A review of plasticity mechanisms that are hypothesized to underlie enhanced recovery from spinal cord injury with stimulation. Frontiers in Molecular Neuroscience. 2020;**13**. Available from: https://www.frontiersin.org/articles/10.3389/fnmol.2020.00163

[45] Grahn PJ, Lavrov IA, Sayenko DG, et al. Enabling task-specific volitional motor functions via spinal cord Neuromodulation in a human with paraplegia. Mayo Clinic Proceedings. 2017;**92**:544-554

[46] Angeli CA, Edgerton VR, Gerasimenko YP, et al. Altering spinal cord excitability enables voluntary movements after chronic complete paralysis in humans. Brain. 2014;**137**:1394-1409

[47] Gill ML, Grahn PJ, Calvert JS, et al. Neuromodulation of lumbosacral spinal networks enables independent stepping after complete paraplegia. Nature Medicine. 2018;**24**:1677-1682

[48] Angeli CA, Boakye M, Morton RA, et al. Recovery of over-ground walking after chronic motor complete spinal cord injury. The New England Journal of Medicine. 2018;**379**:1244-1250

[49] Wagner FB, Mignardot J-B, Le Goff-Mignardot CG, et al. Targeted neurotechnology restores walking in humans with spinal cord injury. Nature. 2018;**563**:65-71

[50] Rowald A, Komi S, Demesmaeker R, et al. Activity-dependent spinal cord neuromodulation rapidly restores trunk and leg motor functions after complete paralysis. Nature Medicine. 2022;**28**:260-271

[51] Alam M, Garcia-Alias G, Jin B, et al. Electrical neuromodulation of the cervical spinal cord facilitates forelimb skilled function recovery in spinal cord injured rats. Experimental Neurology. 2017;**291**:141-150

[52] Lu DC, Edgerton VR, Modaber M, et al. Engaging cervical spinal cord networks to Reenable volitional control of hand function in tetraplegic patients. Neurorehabilitation and Neural Repair. 2016;**30**:951-962

[53] Martin R. Utility and feasibility of transcutaneous spinal cord stimulation for patients with incomplete SCI in therapeutic settings: A review of topic. Frontiers in Rehabilitation Sciences. 2021;**2**. Available from: https://www.frontiersin.org/articles/10.3389/fresc.2021.724003

[54] Taccola G, Sayenko D, Gad P, et al. And yet it moves: Recovery of volitional control after spinal cord injury. Progress in Neurobiology. 2018;**160**:64-81

[55] Meyer C, Hofstoetter US, Hubli M, et al. Immediate effects of transcutaneous spinal cord stimulation on motor function in chronic, sensorimotor incomplete spinal cord injury. Journal of Clinical Medicine. 2020;**9**:1-18. Epub ahead of print. DOI: 10.3390/jcm9113541

[56] Rath M, Vette AH, Ramasubramaniam S, et al. Trunk stability enabled by noninvasive spinal electrical stimulation after spinal cord injury. Journal of Neurotrauma. 2018;**35**:2540-2553

[57] Shapkova EY, Pismennaya EV, Emelyannikov DV, et al. Exoskeleton walk training in paralyzed individuals benefits from transcutaneous lumbar cord tonic electrical stimulation. Frontiers in Neuroscience. 2020;**14**:416

[58] Alam M, Ling YT, Wong AYL, et al. Reversing 21 years of chronic paralysis via non-invasive spinal cord neuromodulation: A case study. Annals of Clinical Translational Neurology. 2020;**7**:829-838

[59] McHugh LV, Miller AA, Leech KA, et al. Feasibility and utility of transcutaneous spinal cord stimulation combined with walking-based therapy

for people with motor incomplete spinal cord injury. Spinal Cord Series And Cases. 2020;**6**:104

[60] Estes S, Zarkou A, Hope JM, et al. Combined transcutaneous spinal stimulation and locomotor training to improve walking function and reduce spasticity in subacute spinal cord injury: A randomized study of clinical feasibility and efficacy. Journal of Clinical Medicine. 2021;**10**:1-17. Epub ahead of print. DOI: 10.3390/jcm10061167

[61] Freyvert Y, Yong NA, Morikawa E, et al. Engaging cervical spinal circuitry with non-invasive spinal stimulation and buspirone to restore hand function in chronic motor complete patients. Scientific Reports. 2018;**8**:15546

[62] Inanici F, Brighton LN, Samejima S, et al. Transcutaneous spinal cord stimulation restores hand and arm function after spinal cord injury. IEEE Transactions on Neural Systems and Rehabilitation Engineering a Publications IEEE Engineering Medicine Biology Society. 2021;**29**:310-319

[63] Luo S, Xu H, Zuo Y, et al. A review of functional electrical stimulation treatment in spinal cord injury. Neuromolecular Medicine. 2020;**22**:447-463

[64] van der Scheer JW, Goosey-Tolfrey VL, Valentino SE, et al. Functional electrical stimulation cycling exercise after spinal cord injury: A systematic review of health and fitness-related outcomes. Journal of Neuroengineering and Rehabilitation. 2021;**18**:99

[65] Ibitoye MO, Hamzaid NA, Hasnan N, et al. Strategies for rapid muscle fatigue reduction during FES exercise in individuals with spinal cord injury: A systematic review. PLoS One. 2016;**11**:e0149024

[66] Martin R, Sadowsky C, Obst K, et al. Functional electrical stimulation in spinal cord injury:: From theory to practice. Top Spinal Cord Injury Rehabilitation. 2012;**18**:28-33

[67] Bekhet AH, Bochkezanian V, Saab IM, et al. The effects of electrical stimulation parameters in managing spasticity after spinal cord injury: A systematic review. American Journal of Physical Medicine & Rehabilitation. 2019;**98**:484-499

[68] Yaşar E, Yılmaz B, Göktepe S, et al. The effect of functional electrical stimulation cycling on late functional improvement in patients with chronic incomplete spinal cord injury. Spinal Cord. 2015;**53**:866-869

[69] Thorsen R, Dalla Costa D, Chiaramonte S, et al. A noninvasive Neuroprosthesis augments hand grasp force in individuals with cervical spinal cord injury: The functional and therapeutic effects. Scientific World Journal. 2013;**2013**:836959

[70] Chesterton LS, Lewis AM, Sim J, et al. Transcutaneous electrical nerve stimulation as adjunct to primary care management for tennis elbow: Pragmatic randomised controlled trial (TATE trial). British Journal of Sports Medicine. 2014;**48**:1458 LP 1458

[71] Gossrau G, Wähner M, Kuschke M, et al. Microcurrent transcutaneous electric nerve stimulation in painful diabetic neuropathy: A randomized placebo-controlled study. Pain Medicine. 2011;**12**:953-960

[72] Chen C-C, Johnson MI, McDonough S, et al. The effect of transcutaneous electrical nerve stimulation on local and distal cutaneous blood flow following a prolonged heat stimulus in healthy subjects. Clinical

Physiology and Functional Imaging. 2007;**27**:154-161

[73] Sluka KA, Walsh D. Transcutaneous electrical nerve stimulation: Basic science mechanisms and clinical effectiveness. The Journal of Pain. 2003;**4**:109-121

[74] Mokhtari T, Ren Q, Li N, et al. Transcutaneous electrical nerve stimulation in relieving neuropathic pain: Basic mechanisms and clinical applications. Current Pain and Headache Reports. 2020;**24**:14

[75] Yang Y, Tang Y, Qin H, et al. Efficacy of transcutaneous electrical nerve stimulation in people with pain after spinal cord injury: A meta-analysis. Spinal Cord. 2022;**60**:375-381

[76] Mills PB, Dossa F. Transcutaneous electrical nerve stimulation for Management of Limb Spasticity: A systematic review. American Journal of Physical Medicine & Rehabilitation. 2016;**95**:309-318

[77] Mahmood A, Veluswamy SK, Hombali A, et al. Effect of transcutaneous electrical nerve stimulation on spasticity in adults with stroke: A systematic review and meta-analysis. Archives of Physical Medicine and Rehabilitation. 2019;**100**:751-768

[78] Oo WM. Efficacy of addition of transcutaneous electrical nerve stimulation to standardized physical therapy in subacute spinal spasticity: A randomized controlled trial. Archives of Physical Medicine and Rehabilitation. 2014;**95**:2013-2020

[79] Ping Ho Chung B, Kam Kwan Cheng B. Immediate effect of transcutaneous electrical nerve stimulation on spasticity in patients with spinal cord injury. Clinical Rehabilitation. 2010;**24**:202-210

[80] Sivaramakrishnan A, Solomon JM, Manikandan N. Comparison of transcutaneous electrical nerve stimulation (TENS) and functional electrical stimulation (FES) for spasticity in spinal cord injury - a pilot randomized cross-over trial. The Journal of Spinal Cord Medicine. 2018;**41**:397-406

[81] Jensen MP, Truitt AR, Schomer KG, et al. Frequency and age effects of secondary health conditions in individuals with spinal cord injury: A scoping review. Spinal Cord. 2013;**51**:882-892

[82] Sezer N, Akkuş S, Uğurlu FG. Chronic complications of spinal cord injury. World Journal of Orthopedics. 2015;**6**:24-33

[83] Booth FW, Roberts CK, Laye MJ. Lack of exercise is a major cause of chronic diseases. Comprehensive Physiology. 2012;**2**:1143-1211

[84] Ditunno PL, Patrick M, Stineman M, et al. Who wants to walk? Preferences for recovery after SCI: A longitudinal and cross-sectional study. Spinal Cord. 2008;**46**:500-506

[85] Bruni MF, Melegari C, De Cola MC, et al. What does best evidence tell us about robotic gait rehabilitation in stroke patients: A systematic review and meta-analysis. Journal of Clinical Neuroscience Official Journal of Neurosurgery Society Australas. 2018;**48**:11-17

[86] Carpino G, Pezzola A, Urbano M, et al. Assessing effectiveness and costs in robot-mediated lower limbs rehabilitation: A meta-analysis and state of the art. Journal of Healthcare Engineering. 2018;**2018**:7492024

[87] Nam KY, Kim HJ, Kwon BS, et al. Robot-assisted gait training (Lokomat) improves walking function and

activity in people with spinal cord injury: A systematic review. Journal of Neuroengineering and Rehabilitation. 2017;**14**:24

[88] Contreras-Vidal JL, Bhagat NA, Brantley J, et al. Powered exoskeletons for bipedal locomotion after spinal cord injury. Journal of Neural Engineering. 2016;**13**:31001

[89] Duan R, Qu M, Yuan Y, et al. Clinical benefit of rehabilitation training in spinal cord injury: A systematic review and meta-analysis. Spine (Phila Pa 1976). 2021;**46**:E398-E410

[90] Mehrholz J, Harvey LA, Thomas S, et al. Is body-weight-supported treadmill training or robotic-assisted gait training superior to overground gait training and other forms of physiotherapy in people with spinal cord injury? A systematic review. Spinal Cord. 2017;**55**:722-729

[91] Holanda LJ, Silva PMM, Amorim TC, et al. Robotic assisted gait as a tool for rehabilitation of individuals with spinal cord injury: A systematic review. Journal of Neuroengineering and Rehabilitation. 2017;**14**:126

[92] Rodríguez-Fernández A, Lobo-Prat J, Font-Llagunes JM. Systematic review on wearable lower-limb exoskeletons for gait training in neuromuscular impairments. Journal of Neuroengineering and Rehabilitation. 2021;**18**:22

[93] Colombo G, Joerg M, Schreier R, et al. Treadmill training of paraplegic patients using a robotic orthosis. Journal of Rehabilitation Research and Development. 2000;**37**:693-700

[94] Donati ARC, Shokur S, Morya E, et al. Long-term training with a brain-machine Interface-based gait protocol induces partial neurological recovery in paraplegic patients. Scientific Reports. 2016;**6**:30383

[95] Aach M, Cruciger O, Sczesny-Kaiser M, et al. Voluntary driven exoskeleton as a new tool for rehabilitation in chronic spinal cord injury: A pilot study. The Spine Journal. 2014;**14**:2847-2853

[96] Cragg JJ, Noonan VK, Krassioukov A, et al. Cardiovascular disease and spinal cord injury: Results from a national population health survey. Neurology. 2013;**81**:723-728

[97] Garshick E, Kelley A, Cohen SA, et al. A prospective assessment of mortality in chronic spinal cord injury. Spinal Cord. 2005;**43**:408-416

[98] Ozgurtas T, Alaca R, Gulec M, et al. Do spinal cord injuries adversely affect serum lipoprotein profiles? Military Medicine. 2003;**168**:545-547

[99] Hollis BC, Lafavor JD, Mauder V, et al. Inflammation and insulin sensitivity In spinal cord injured subjects: 761: May 28 2: 00 PM-2: 15 PM. Medicine & Science in Sports Exercise. 2009;**41**:73

[100] Krassioukov A, Eng JJ, Warburton DE, et al. A systematic review of the management of orthostatic hypotension after spinal cord injury. Archives of Physical Medicine and Rehabilitation. 2009;**90**:876-885

[101] Claydon VE, Steeves JD, Krassioukov A. Orthostatic hypotension following spinal cord injury: Understanding clinical pathophysiology. Spinal Cord. 2006;**44**:341-351

[102] Krassioukov A, Warburton DE, Teasell R, et al. A systematic review of the management of autonomic Dysreflexia after spinal cord injury. Archives of Physical Medicine and Rehabilitation. 2009;**90**:682-695

[103] Blackmer J. Rehabilitation medicine: 1. Autonomic dysreflexia. Canadian Medical Association Journal = J l'Association medicale Can. 2003;**169**:931-935

[104] Krassioukov AV, Furlan JC, Fehlings MG. Autonomic dysreflexia in acute spinal cord injury: An under-recognized clinical entity. Journal of Neurotrauma. 2003;**20**:707-716

[105] Cardozo CP. Respiratory complications of spinal cord injury. The Journal of Spinal Cord Medicine. 2007;**30**:307-308

[106] Brown R, DiMarco AF, Hoit JD, et al. Respiratory dysfunction and management in spinal cord injury. Respiratory Care. 2006;**51**:853-870

[107] Tamplin J, Berlowitz DJ. A systematic review and meta-analysis of the effects of respiratory muscle training on pulmonary function in tetraplegia. Spinal Cord. 2014;**52**:175-180

[108] Van Houtte S, Vanlandewijck Y, Gosselink R. Respiratory muscle training in persons with spinal cord injury: A systematic review. Respiratory Medicine. 2006;**100**:1886-1895

[109] Shin JC, Han EY, Cho KH, et al. Improvement in pulmonary function with short-term rehabilitation treatment in spinal cord injury patients. Scientific Reports. 2019;**9**:17091

[110] Park J, Choi WA, Kang S-W. Pulmonary rehabilitation in high cervical spinal cord injury: A series of 133 consecutive cases. Spinal Cord. Epub ahead of print. 2022;**60**:1014-1019 DOI: 10.1038/s41393-022-00816-8

[111] Postma K, Haisma JA, de Groot S, et al. Changes in pulmonary function during the early years after inpatient rehabilitation in persons with spinal cord injury: A prospective cohort study. Archives of Physical Medicine and Rehabilitation. 2013;**94**:1540-1546

[112] Sheel AW, Reid WD, Townson AF, et al. Effects of exercise training and inspiratory muscle training in spinal cord injury: A systematic review. The Journal of Spinal Cord Medicine. 2008;**31**:500-508

[113] Berlowitz DJ, Tamplin J. Respiratory muscle training for cervical spinal cord injury. Cochrane Database of Systematic Reviews. 2013;**2013**. Epub ahead of print. DOI: 10.1002/14651858.CD008507.pub2

[114] Kuris EO, Alsoof D, Osorio C, et al. Bowel and bladder Care in Patients with Spinal Cord Injury. JAAOS – Journal of American Academic Orthopedic Surgery. 2022;**30**:263-272. Available from: https://journals.lww.com/jaaos/Fulltext/2022/03150/Bowel_and_Bladder_Care_in_Patients_With_Spinal.5.aspx

[115] Cardenas DD, Hoffman JM, Kirshblum S, et al. Etiology and incidence of rehospitalization after traumatic spinal cord injury: A multicenter analysis. Archives of Physical Medicine and Rehabilitation. 2004;**85**:1757-1763

[116] Tate DG, Wheeler T, Lane GI, et al. Recommendations for evaluation of neurogenic bladder and bowel dysfunction after spinal cord injury and/or disease. The Journal of Spinal Cord Medicine. 2020;**43**:141-164

[117] Zlatev DV, Shem K, Elliott CS. How many spinal cord injury patients can catheterize their own bladder? The epidemiology of upper extremity function as it affects bladder management. Spinal Cord. 2016;**54**:287-291

[118] Savic G, Frankel HL, Jamous MA, et al. Long-term bladder and bowel

management after spinal cord injury: A 20-year longitudinal study. Spinal Cord. 2018;**56**:575-581

[119] Emmanuel A. Neurogenic bowel dysfunction. F1000Research. 2019;**8**. Epub ahead of print. DOI: 10.12688/f1000research.20529.1

[120] Johns JS, Krogh K, Ethans K, et al. Pharmacological Management of Neurogenic Bowel Dysfunction after spinal cord injury and multiple sclerosis: A systematic review and clinical implications. Journal of Clinical Medicine. 2021;**10**:1-15. Epub ahead of print. DOI: 10.3390/jcm10040882

[121] Coggrave M, Norton C, Wilson-Barnett J. Management of neurogenic bowel dysfunction in the community after spinal cord injury: A postal survey in the United Kingdom. Spinal Cord. 2009;**47**:323

[122] Stoffel JT, Van der Aa F, Wittmann D, et al. Neurogenic bowel management for the adult spinal cord injury patient. World Journal of Urology. 2018;**36**:1587-1592

[123] Finnerup NB, Johannesen IL, Sindrup SH, et al. Pain and dysesthesia in patients with spinal cord injury: A postal survey. Spinal Cord. 2001;**39**:256-262

[124] Jensen MP, Chodroff MJ, Dworkin RH. The impact of neuropathic pain on health-related quality of life: Review and implications. Neurology. 2007;**68**:1178-1182

[125] Putzke JD, Richards SJ, Hicken BL, et al. Interference due to pain following spinal cord injury: Important predictors and impact on quality of life. Pain. 2002;**100**:231-242

[126] Siddall PJ, McClelland JM, Rutkowski SB, et al. A longitudinal study of the prevalence and characteristics of pain in the first 5 years following spinal cord injury. Pain. 2003;**103**:249-257

[127] Bryce TN, Biering-Sørensen F, Finnerup NB, et al. International spinal cord injury pain classification: Part I. background and description. Spinal Cord. 2012;**50**:413-417

[128] Burke D, Fullen BM, Stokes D, et al. Neuropathic pain prevalence following spinal cord injury: A systematic review and meta-analysis. European Journal of Pain. 2017;**21**:29-44

[129] Hatch MN, Cushing TR, Carlson GD, et al. Neuropathic pain and SCI: Identification and treatment strategies in the 21st century. Journal of the Neurological Sciences. 2018;**384**:75-83

[130] Adams MM, Hicks AL. Spasticity after spinal cord injury. Spinal Cord. 2005;**43**:577-586

[131] Holtz KA, Lipson R, Noonan VK, et al. Prevalence and effect of problematic spasticity after traumatic spinal cord injury. Archives of Physical Medicine and Rehabilitation. 2017;**98**:1132-1138

[132] Anson CA, Shepherd C. Incidence of secondary complications in spinal cord injury. International Journal of Rehabilitation Research Internationale Zeitschrift fur Rehabilitations fors Review International Rech Readapt. 1996;**19**:55-66

[133] Taricco M, Pagliacci MC, Telaro E, et al. Pharmacological interventions for spasticity following spinal cord injury: Results of a Cochrane systematic review. Europa Medicophysica. 2006;**42**:5-15

[134] Khurana SR, Garg DS. Spasticity and the use of intrathecal baclofen in patients with spinal cord injury. Physical Medicine and Rehabilitation Clinics of North America. 2014;**25**:655-669. ix